The Boy Wh  Trees

by

Sian Bezuidenhout

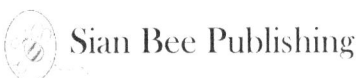 Sian Bee Publishing

To my father, Eddie Pather

My favourite storyteller

Published in the United Kingdom in 2018 by Sian Bee Publishing

Content copyright @ Sian Bezuidenhout, 2018

All rights reserved. No portion of this book may be reproduced, stored in a retrieval system or transmitted at any time by or any means mechanical, electronic, photocopying, recording or otherwise, without the prior, written permission of the publisher.

The right of Sian Bezuidenhout to be identified as the author of this work has been asserted by her in accordance with the Copyright, Designs and Patents act, 1988.

First printed August 2018.

This is a work of fiction. Names, characters, places, incidents and dialogues are products of the author's imagination or are used fictitiously. Any resemblance to actual people, living or dead, events or locales is entirely coincidental.

The few organizations/ characters drawn from real life are specifically mentioned and acknowledged in the book.

This book is not intended as a substitute for therapeutic or medical intervention.

ISBN 978-1-9164588-0-2

Introduction

I am a tree ambassador. A landscape looney aka lunatic. I have always been drawn to trees.

These statuesque, majestic creatures magically transform every landscape. They work so hard for us, giving us their souls in the process.

A bit of technical information:

Like all plants, trees absorb carbon dioxide through their leaves. They then turn it into sugar during photosynthesis, which helps them grow. They release oxygen which animals breathe in, so trees help to keep us alive. In addition, trees reduce climate change. Carbon dioxide is a greenhouse gas which stops heat leaving the earth's atmosphere, thus keeping the earth warmer than it would be otherwise. By removing this carbon dioxide and locking it away, trees help to reduce global warming. During deforestation, trees are cut down, or killed, leaving fewer trees to do the job of removing carbon dioxide from the atmosphere. When the trees are burnt, the stored carbon is released into the atmosphere helping to create the greenhouse effect.

This has a major impact on the earth's ability to sustain life. Algae die in warm temperatures and small fish that feed on them therefore die too, thus creating a ripple effect in the food chain. There are many more negative ripples from temperatures rising, like how it interferes with the rhythms of life: hibernation, mating, natural habitats and so on.

We need to act. For if we cut down all the forests, what kind of planet do we have? One that will not sustain life as we know it. So that is how humanity will finally end.

There are also other environmental benefits to trees that we lose when they are cut down. They offer homes to animals, birds, insects, micro-organisms and even people. They provide food, storage, protection, comfort and love. They sustain entire ecosystems. Some, like me, believe they have their own unique language and communicate to those who believe in them.

I'm not just some sad eco-warrior fixating on this crucial topic.

I speak to trees.

I don't just hug them, I whisper to them. And they whisper back. I want to help them, the way they help me.

My name is Alan Arbour. My name alone speaks of a strange, unmistakable connection to trees. And I don't care if it makes people uncomfortable to know this.

You see, trees have helped me heal. I have a pervasive, neurobiological, developmental disability called Asperger's syndrome. I prefer to call myself an Aspie. This is my story.

Alan

Alan

Chapter 1

Once upon a time, I lived in a two up and two down with my mum and dad. Dad was a painter and decorator, mum was a dressmaker. We had a simple but easy life. I was happy. So happy. My room was at the top, it was a large, light space overlooking the back garden with its patch of emerald green grass and colourful flowers on the sides. The decoration was perfect, my parents didn't change it. Against a pale cream background, tall trees rose up revealing branches of nesting birds, it really was quite fascinating. You could lie there for ages, with your hands behind your head, just watching the scene, imagining yourself there, in the forest. The detail was staggering, I picked out the veins on the leaves, the peeling bark on the trunk, the glorious purple and green plumage of the birds sitting on eggs on the high branches. It was expensive wallpaper, thick and glossy and vibrant.

The main word in my house at the time was 'busy.' Mum took orders for bespoke, fancy prom dresses. She was so good that she had a steady supply of customers just from word of mouth. She was clueless about computers, otherwise she could have sold the dresses online. As it was, people would come knocking to have fittings done and to collect their dresses, the house was full of voices. Off cuts of fabric, buttons, sequins and other accessories lay in their individual boxes on a shelf that we were never allowed to touch. The noisy drone of the sewing machine created a constant backdrop. I'm usually uncomfortable with loud noises but for some reason, I felt joyful in that house.

Mum took me everywhere with her. She would push me in the pram around with her to shops that sold supplies, there'd be rows and rows of patterns in paper pouches with colour pictures on the cover showing what the dresses were meant to look like.

They were accessorised with hats, belts, crystals and shawls. Mum would talk me through them, asking me to indicate whether one was better than the next. Of course, she was just talking to herself, thinking out loud so to speak, but I didn't mind, I loved to be part of her world. Sometimes, she'd slip the inside sleeve out, spread it on the large table and examine it, discussing it with the shop assistant. If she could change the sleeves it would work better, or with the other pattern, the shoulders looked too heavy with the pads, could she tweak that bit? Then, she'd sit at the table, poring over boxes and boxes of little colourful buttons, zips, motifs, crystals and sequins, carefully selecting the right combination for her designs. I noticed everything with a satisfied smug. She said that I didn't communicate much. But I picked up everything.

As an only child, I nestled in the bosom of my parent's love, enjoying their attention exclusively. My heart must have lit up with all the love in that house, even though I didn't show emotion easily. Mum said that I was passive. I didn't reach out for cuddles and I didn't cry much. I slept a lot, ate well and seemed to like being by myself.

She was beautiful, dad told her that every day. With her shoulder length dark hair, creamy, flawless skin and chocolate coloured eyes, she got looked at everywhere we went. She laughed a lot too, throwing back her head in that way of hers, revealing sparkling white teeth and full red lips.

Her sewing room was also the living room, and every evening she tried to tidy things away so that we could eat and watch TV together. Sometimes when she had several orders on the go, she didn't stop, working all day and most of the night. Once, Dad found her slumped at her sewing machine in the morning.

Dad was a painter and decorator, most times I'd hear him on the phone saying that he was too busy to take on more work. 'I'm rushed off my feet,' he'd say to new customers, checking his work schedules in his little black diary, 'but I'll see what I can do.'

Then, he'd say to mom, 'Never turn away work when you have a family to feed!' and they'd both scoop me up in a bear hug. I loved those hugs, which child doesn't? Dad smelled of mints which he chewed constantly to disguise the fact that he smoked, Mum smelled of something sweet and flowery. And I smelled of baby.

Just before I turned five, dad fell off an extra tall ladder at work and the equipment fell on him. He was a tall, skinny man, basically a bigger version of me. He fell onto his arm and broke it. In hospital, he also complained of crippling back pain, something that would never really go away from that day on. He stopped work and lay in bed for months, leaving a sad, sour atmosphere in the house. Mum would pop up and down with trays of toast, soup and cups of tea until she too gave up because it became too much for her.

'How am I going to pay the bills all on my own?' she'd ask her sister Auntie Linda tearfully, during her nightly phone calls. 'I can't look after Alan, take him to school and back, see customers, make clothes, cook, clean and run up and down with trays of food for him. Something has to give, I can't carry on!'

When gran died, she left the house to her two daughters, Auntie Linda and mum. My parents took a bank loan to pay off Auntie Linda and we kept the house for ourselves. Auntie lived in Hampshire, with her husband, Uncle Ali. It was too expensive for us to go to visit them, so every few months, she took the train to London and came over to the house to see us. We loved seeing her, she always brought flowers, chocolates and a bottle of wine. There'd be a toy for me too, something with a sound or lights. Everyone said that I was too absorbed in my own world, I needed to interact more. But, to me, the world was perfect as it was. You could feel the love in our house.

But everything stopped when dad got sick. The flow of money in the house stopped. Mum refused to work, saying that it was all too much for her. The letters demanding money came thick and fast. The bank, the electricity and gas company, the water company, the shops that my parents had opened accounts in.

Mum would fetch me from school and usher me to a surprisingly still, quiet house. It smelled of something stale and sad. Instead of cake and hot chocolate for snack, she'd serve me bread and butter with weak tea. When I refused, she'd smack me, then cry and send me to my room, where I'd lie in shock, listening to my dad crying in pain. The wallpaper sustained me, kept me glued. The trees beckoned.

'Don't worry,' they whispered. 'Everything will be okay.'

In no time, we sold the house and paid the bills, leaving nothing left over. Gone was my beautiful room with the trees and birds. Gone was my mum's sewing stuff which she had to sell. And gone was dad, after a massive row about where we would live next.

The council could only offer us temporary accommodation at first, in a shared hostel, with three other people on our floor. Looking at them, I was so scared that, at six, I started to wet the bed again, which got me smacks and groundings in that new, little cupboard of a room that they gave me. There was Max, an old man covered in grey hair, who smelled strongly of alcohol and talked constantly to himself about the war. I feared his wild looking glass eye. Once, in the shared kitchen, he saluted me, then said loudly, 'Reporting for duty Sir!' I had to keep my eye on him, while I buttered my toast. Didn't want him leaping up and grabbing a knife, thinking that I was the enemy.

Then there was David, a shifty looking middle- aged man who kept trying to put his arm around mum. He'd just come out of prison and he kept talking about 'doing deals' on the phone. I liked it when he got me bars of chocolate, all for the chance of passing his love letters to mum. I'd polish the chocolate off in my room, then read the silly little notes before placing them in my school bag so that I could throw them in the school bin. Lastly there was someone that no one knew much about, he just sat in the shared living space, rocking and crying. When he saw us, he'd make a beeline for his room where he'd continue, I know, I stood outside once, listening.

Time flew by. It felt like we'd been in that hellish place for months. When I asked about my dad, mum would sigh and shrug her shoulders. She still wore her wedding ring and the locket with his picture inside, around her neck. But I went on and on about dad. I just wanted everything back to normal. It was only about a year later, when we moved into our two bedroomed council house, that she told me that dad was in prison for robbery and assault and that they had divorced.

Three years later, she died and my whole world came crumbling down.

Chapter 2

Lemon. The fruity, sweet, aroma filled the apartment making the boy salivate. There were other notes too. Herbs, roasted garlic, butter. In a trance, he followed the scent of food, turning from the cluttered hallway into the shabby living room and then into the small, narrow kitchen which was usually bare. Until now. On the table, a large, golden, roast chicken nestled in an oven tray surrounded by crispy potatoes. Next to it was a baked chocolate pudding in the shape of a volcano, on one side, it had started to ooze leaving a molten chocolate trail, like lava. The maddening smell of butter and chocolate made him want to reach out and eat it with his fingers, he was so hungry, his eyes were as big as saucers. His stomach had been growling for food but now....

Bang! Bang!

No, he had to eat first.

Bang, bang, bang!

Oh, what was that nasty sound? And why now, just as he was about to have his first proper meal in years? Slowly, reluctantly, he abandoned the dream and opened his eyes. The old-fashioned phone next to his bed showed him the time. 3.30 am. The middle of the night. He had school in the morning.

With a deep sigh, he roused himself and approached the front door.

'Alan! You there? C'mon open the door boy!'

What would Mrs. Shen, his next-door neighbour think? All this noise in the middle of the night? It just wasn't fair.

With a kind of despair, he unchained and unbolted the door. His father stood there along with a small party of what the boy silently called 'undesirables.' They had probably been drinking in the local pub and then gone on somewhere else to continue the party. Waves of smells, bad ones this time, reached his nose and he tried unsuccessfully to swat them away without appearing rude. If he was outwardly hostile to his father's down-and-out friends, he was sure to get a slap, especially when his father was drunk, like now. The stench of cigarette smoke mixed with alcohol clung to his father's clothes as he burst inside, pushing by the sleepy boy, the others followed, hooting with laughter. Someone with teeth as yellow as corn kernels pulled a bottle of drink and a packet of something foul smelling out of his jacket pocket and smiled at him. Sensitive to smells, Alan felt his stomach recoil. Angrily, he went back in to his narrow, dark bedroom muttering something about the selfishness of people. It would take him a long, long time to fall back into sleep now. There was no chance that he could get that food dream back, not with the carry on in the living room now.

'Stupid boy!' he heard. 'Worried about getting up for school.' Laughter.

'School is for losers!'

'When I was that age, I was out all night.'

'He never learns anything anyway. He's always in his own world. Don't know why anyone like that would want to bother with school!'

Alan lay in bed, trying to get the dream back, wishing he was somewhere else.

Alan

Chapter 3

When I grow up, I want to work for the Woodland Trust. The website says that it's:

'The UK's largest woodland conservation charity.' They go on to explain that they protect and safeguard woods currently at risk, they restore ancient woodlands and they also create new, native woodland. I'm blown away by their passion for woodland conservation and want desperately to be part of something as fulfilling as this.

I'm not a germophobe, but sometimes closed spaces make me feel suffocated. Imagine all the germs in the air in a closed classroom, and all the students in the room breathing this in. No, that thought makes me anxious and slightly sick! I'd rather be in an oxygen rich environment, like in a forest, where I can breathe fresh, clean air and feel energized.

I've researched the therapeutic effects of walking amongst trees thoroughly, so I know that I'm on the right track with my tree fixation. Ever heard of 'forest bathing?' The Japanese call it 'Shinrin-Yoku'. Basically, they believe that each time you walk around in a living forest, you receive a kind of therapy which can lift your mood, help you to sleep better and generally support you in functioning more effectively. As an Aspie with a bunch of needs, I don't need to spell out how crucial this natural therapy is for me. The best part is that it's free. When I've felt pent up and angry in the past, trees have helped to de-escalate my anxiety. They have an instant, calming effect on me.

I could become a tree photographer. At school, Sir says that my Photography grades are the highest in the class.

'For someone who is disabled, you have an uncanny gift for capturing the poetry of nature,' he says. He also says that gadgets are my thing. That's probably why I'm so good with cameras.

He refuses to call me Special Needs. He says that it's a condescending label created by an 'ablest mindset.' I can just about understand this, it's like saying that I'm suboptimal as a human being, as defined by people who think that *they* are optimal or normal. So, instead of seeing me as unique, they would see me as being flawed. Sir said that everyone was special, that we all had strengths and weaknesses, peaks and troughs. I wasn't so good around people, but others were not so good around gadgets. I appreciated Sir's support, he believed in me. That's why I did so well in his class. Photography was my best subject. When I was bored, I always went back there to finish my work or just to put in extra time.

I could spend ages taking pictures and developing them in the dark room, seeing the image transform before my very eyes was so magical. Pity I don't have a camera at home. If only I had a camera, or my bike was fixed...I'd have more options about how to spend my spare time. I have oodles and poodles of time on my hands and lots of ideas.

My whole life, I've been different. Overwhelmingly different. But my combination or cocktail of special needs did not come with an owner's manual. Who would have thought about putting dyslexia, dyspraxia, ADHD, and Asperger's together in one impossible mix? Whew! No wonder teachers run when they see me coming. Assistants too, most of them. Nowadays, teachers are judged by the government on how successful they are at teaching us, if we don't show that we are making progress then they are seen to be crap, maybe their jobs will be on the line.

'Substandard! You're a substandard teacher!'

No one deserves that, it's so cruel. Why can't we just be recognized for what we can do, as opposed to what we can't do? It's not the teachers' fault that

I'm difficult. It's not my fault either. It is what it is. I'm not asking anyone to fix me, I just want to be accepted for what I am, warts and all.

I don't like complaining about my life too much. I've had a few key life lessons, blessings if you like. One of those is the systematic bullying that I've experienced all the way from primary school. I say systematic as it's pretty much been non- stop. They picked on my name (Alan, but then, who calls their kid Alan?), my learning difficulties, my deprived home environment, my aggressive personality, my unfashionable clothes, my alcoholic mother, my jailbird father, my free school meals and my silences in classes where social interaction was expected. Of course, I was withdrawn. I'm high functioning, not dumb, I see things. Beyond what is actually there. Call it a fine- tuned perception or an acute ability to read and predict from situations brought on by my painful home life. Which kid has to budget, buy food and cook at primary school age?

But I digress as usual.

I was talking about how bullying can be a gift. You see, it became a norm, a daily expectation. And after a while, the magic hand of time was the best therapy. I became habituated over time, developed a thick skin, words washed over me, just skimming over me, not getting embedded into my psyche. I had learned how to cope with adversity. Ignore and move on. Fast forward. So, while they were busy laughing and poking fun at me like the way they treated freaks in those absurd Victorian circuses, I just blocked them out and focused on something positive, like trees. Studying them, photographing them, even talking to them.

Unbeknown to teachers, I can read. I read very well. Otherwise why would I have stacks and stacks of books at the side of my bed, in fact all around my bed? Okay most are about trees but still. I just don't like reading about things that don't interest me, like most of the books that teachers force you to read. Another thing, I'm a control freak. You'll never be able to force me to do anything I don't want to do. So, I don't read or write in class, it's so boring. I pick and choose what I want to do. I want to be in the driving seat. Always. If anyone pushes me to the edge, they're triggering a violent outburst that shocks even hardcore naughty kids. When I erupt, it's not a pretty sight.

To be honest, I enjoy one to one support, which deprived child doesn't? All that attention. Support assistants tend to be just the right side of nurturing and matronly and I appreciate that. Mother substitutes. I learn quickly with them. I'm high functioning as I said, they know it and they clamour to work with me. I see them fighting over me as they sort out their schedules.

'If I work with Alan on a Monday, maybe you can support him on Tuesday? But wait, what about consistency? Maybe *I* should keep working with him.'

I've learned a lot, I know how to be calm and controlled now. I can self-manage my anxiety or de-escalate my anger. And I can communicate my feelings too, if I sense that it's going to bubble up in me, I just flash my Time Out card and I'm allowed to go to somewhere peaceful for a few minutes, to calm down.

Obviously, I seek refuge in the small grove of trees on the playground, to be amongst the umbrella of green is the most soothing thing. If I had the resources, I'd paint my bedroom leaf green and dot huge plants throughout.

So, I harnessed the bullying to my own advantage, used it to become resilient and unbreakable. In fact, now, I feel sorry for people who don't get the required reaction when they bully me. Because bullies have problems too, or so we're taught. No child or person bullies another without some negative back story hiding somewhere, it's about a quest for power or self-esteem that they're not getting at home I think. So, for example if they are being treated badly at home, they mask their true feelings of being unworthy and express it as acting 'hard' or 'cool' in front of others, they want the applause when they pick on the victim, they crave approval so badly that they will hit, punch and assault that poor, submissive victim. For no reason whatsoever. It could be that you're first in the dinner queue. So, you get shoved and kicked to the back. You could be looking in a certain direction and they don't like it. So, you get slapped. If you're minding your own business in class, they laugh and call you 'stupid' or 'retarded.' Sometimes, they follow you home, calling you names all the way.

I pity bullies, I really do. We need more work on improving their mindsets because otherwise they grow up and continue to bully adults. It's all about learnt patterns of behavior or habituation, as my support teacher told me. She was trying to help me identify trigger factors for when I got anxious and angry, but she covered bullies and victims too. See that's why I've accepted that I have special needs. I see myself as special. I have some amazing people who work with me. Of course, there are lots of not so amazing ones, but I'm not prepared to call them suboptimal. Maybe it's all about the fit. They don't fit with me, I fit with nice, patient, calm and knowledgeable professionals.

I know that my voice shakes, but I speak my truth.

I'll never forget how I found mum.

Chapter 4

'If you can't concentrate on basic work, you really shouldn't be here!' The English teacher was mean. She had a habit of ignoring him or teasing him with her sarcastic remarks. As soon as he entered the classroom, she would roll her tired eyes.

'It's you again. Why can't you be absent?'

Everyone would fall about laughing. He had always experienced problems with reading and writing and many of his secondary school teachers hated him. He was just too much trouble, you had to start from scratch with somebody like him. Clearly, his primary school had not done a good job in preparing him with the basics. He had not mastered phonics. He had not been shown how to shape letters properly or make them sit on the lines. Secondary school was like driving in the fast lane.

Whoosh! There was so much happening. Visiting speakers, competitions, football matches, assembly, assessments, exams and lesson observations. The content of lessons was so sophisticated, you had to keep up, as every week you were supposed to demonstrate advanced skills. No wonder some kids just gave up. It was especially challenging for kids who didn't speak fluent English, or for those with Special Needs. Like him.

'I hope I get sent out!' they'd say before the lesson. 'I don't care where I'm sent to or how they want to punish me, I can't do it!'

Sometimes, he wished that teachers could read kids better and know this. Maybe then, they'd make lessons more fun, and easier to get. Instead, some barely made eye contact with the kids, they kept their eyes fixed on the computer screen on the desk and delivered lessons without even standing up. Some became especially grumpy during observations. It meant that a team leader or inspector came into the classroom to watch the lesson and check that the students were learning. Well, a small cluster of kids was always going to mess it up for everyone. Always. And Alan was in this group. If you took one look at him, you'd see why.

His clothes looked crumpled, his white shirt given free just a few months ago by the uniform shop, now looked yellow. How on earth had he done that? It was unbelievable what children got up to these days! His face looked like he hadn't washed in a long time, there were bits of white around his eyes and dried snot around his nostrils. His fingernails were bitten to the quick and his hands were dirty, so much so that every teacher started with, 'Alan, go wash your hands before you touch your book.' He smelled so bad that other students refused to sit next to him or accept him in group work. Drama was out of the question, he was too frail for team games, too stupid for anything competitive. Teachers would recoil when he approached the desk, asking him to stand far away if he wanted to ask something. So, he stopped asking. In fact, he stopped answering questions, he didn't even answer his name when the register was called. Usually one of the others would call out if it was a new teacher doing the register, 'Alan *is* here, he just doesn't talk.' Most times, he was instructed to leave the class and sit alone, in the library, where he could use the computers to do research. He could check out any topic. Whatever. If he stayed away from others, didn't steal the books or interfere with the librarian when she was busy, he could pretty much look up anything. He could even go for a walk, or leave the school and go elsewhere, to another school where people like him would be welcomed. Here, he was a problem, like a fly that wouldn't leave you alone. So, he became invisible.

Once, before he started studying in the library, a young, keen teaching assistant whisked him away to the Learning Support Department where she made him do some writing, some reading and oddly, some walking around. On her clipboard, she recorded the results of her investigations. Next, she asked him a bunch of questions about his habits and then wrote down a bit more. He had to tell her a lot of things that he never shared with anyone. For example, how he had to do things in threes. Like when he unlocked the door to his flat each day, he had to do it three times. It meant unlocking then locking then unlocking and locking until each set was done three times. At home, he touched his head three times and there were other things that he could only do if it meant that he could do it three times. He liked the shape and form of the number three. It was safe. One was dangerous, it was so close to zero on the number line. If you slipped off, you were a zero, a nothing. He couldn't bear that. Two was the wrong shape, it was too untidy, too squiggly. Eight was perfect, two zeros balanced on top of each other in total harmony. But if he did his rituals eight times each, he'd never be able to leave the house, let alone do all the chores that had landed slowly but surely, on his tender shoulders. So, to compromise, he cut eight in half, making three which also seemed the perfect number, it was balanced, he was safe.

The young assistant had started to become more interested in his case after that. Fixing him with her sharp blue eyes, she asked, pretending to sound casual, what chores he did at home. He was an only child after all, he didn't have to cook and clean for nine siblings unlike other students. Well, he said, his mother was dead. He had found her slumped and stinking of drink in an alleyway. That had been three years ago. Then his dad had been released from prison where he had been banged up for robbery and assault and they had moved to a new flat, in the area around the school. His dad was warm and supportive, he lied. But his important job in the city meant that he came home late so he, Alan, had to clean, take the bins out, and prepare dinner. He didn't mind as he was learning life skills every day.

'So, you are left alone a lot?' he could feel trouble brewing in the air, could picture the ugly sneer on his dad's face when he realized that he'd been snitching.

'No no!' he lied. Lies seemed to roll off his tongue like something slick and slippery, he knew how to keep his hands from twitching and his gaze steady.

'My neighbour looks after me. Dad pays her, and she stays with me until he gets back from his posh job in an office.'

Maybe that was going too far. Most days, you had to visit The Golden Lion pub if you needed to have a meeting with his dad. Some days, he wasn't even there, he just seemed to vanish, only to reappear a few days later like nothing had happened. He lived in that grey tracksuit and his trainers were encrusted with dirt. Nobody used the bathroom in his flat, ever since his dad had started to stockpile stolen goods in the bath, he was not allowed to use it. Besides, bathing was for losers, his dad said. Throughout the week, shifty eyed people would come and go, either delivering more stolen goods or buying. There were car radios, watches, wallets, phones, Sat Navs in boxes and more. He was not allowed to even talk about it, let alone touch the goods. So, he tapped his head three times and walked away.

Eventually, after writing up her report, the assistant gave him a chocolate bar which he devoured in a few gulps. Then, she escorted him back to his English class where she shared her findings in a grave, soft tone which he could hear clearly as he sat in front pretending to read a book. He had so many issues, she didn't know here to start, her report would be coming out later. First off there was the Dyslexia and Dyspraxia. Then the OCD. He was obviously neglected so this meant safeguarding issues. She wanted to oversee his case, he was worth that wasn't he? Every child deserved a chance in life. She would be the one to help him, make sure he had his free school meal each day and more, give him another free uniform, show him where the showers in the PE department were, buy him soap, shampoo and deodorant. It was important to look after children properly, she said, if we didn't we would be failing them, how could he be expected to learn if he didn't have the basics. He was cute and loveable, he had just been through a lot. It meant that she had to take him out of English classes a lot, but it was worth it.

The teacher had to play her part too. There were several tools to support him with his work as he struggled to read and write, and the teacher would have to start using them. She would also have to prepare different lessons just for him as his needs were different to the others.

This was the deal breaker.

He could sense her frustration. Tension hung in the air like a bad smell.

'Oh sure. Listen would you mind watching the class for a bit?'

'No problem, where are you off to?'

'Well, I'm just nipping off home to fetch my sense of humour tablets, I seem to have forgotten them at home.'

Silence.

Luckily the other kids were on laptops, they were meant to be typing up their stories. Alan knew that they were on games that they would quickly minimize if the teacher approached.

'Look, you're going to have to excuse me,' the teacher said, sighing, 'I'm already knackered. Done in! With the behaviour problems, the marking and the lesson preparation for the normal students, I just don't feel like coming to work anymore! It's an overload. Now, you're telling me that:

One. You won't be able to support the other twenty-nine students with *their* needs, instead, you're planning to make it your life's mission to focus on just the one student!' She rolled her eyes. 'You know the class. If they're not on laptops, they'd be climbing on the windowsills! Or worse, setting the place on fire! You're not employed here just to save one student, you're here because I told the Principal that I needed help with the behaviour of the whole class! If it wasn't for me, you wouldn't have a job!

Two. It's not your job to tell me to prepare separate lessons for Alan. I know what I can manage and what I can't. And anyone who gives me pressure over this extra duty, well, they may have to see the back of me. I might just go on a long, long leave of absence for stress reasons. They'd have to pay me just to stay at home. I know my rights. Don't they send these kids to places where they can help them? He doesn't fit in here, just look at him! He's not even reading; the book is upside down! I'm on the edge as it is. I have problems at home. Any more and I'm leaving. If I so much as hear a whisper of a lesson observation, I'll just walk out that door and never come back, they can find someone else to teach these…'

The teacher's face had started to twitch with tension. Her eyeballs looked like they were popping out. Alan watched her, terrified that she would fizz and pop during her meltdown.

'Just er, just take him to the library, he can work there each lesson. It's a quiet environment, he can look at the pictures in the books, play games on the computer, that sort of thing,' she said eventually. 'I never want to see him again. And you, I need you here, your job is to help these other students, they too deserve our support.'

Alan

Chapter 5

I suffer from anxiety attacks and I'm hypersensitive. A riot of colour confuses me, gives me a headache. I can't breathe. So, I prefer monochromatic tones, which means black and white. Except of course when it comes to trees, who can turn away from the visually breathtaking sight of oaks or maple trees in autumn? All that yellow, orange and gold! I'd love to go to Maine in New England USA, for example, as the place seems to be a prime example of how trees dress differently to suit the seasons. But I also know that hordes of visitors flock there every year to see the dramatic autumnal scenes, they call it fall there of course. So, I can't really go. I'm allergic to crowds. Can't think, just want to scream and lash out. Being crushed is not something I ever want to experience.

I am a control freak obsessed with the number three. But I'm not in control when mum drinks. In fact, I'm full of fear. Will she come home? What state will she be in? Will she be ill? Who could I call to help us? Is she safe wherever she is?

She never used to be like this. Slowly, over the years, she let her obsession with dad take over, she gained weight, stopped sewing and lost her passion for living. The man was a jailbird. Crime had become a habit. There was no point in pining for him! He just came out and went back in again. How could she lose interest in life just because of someone like that? I pondered over this non-stop. Because effectively, in throwing away her life, she was throwing *me* away too. She morphed into someone I couldn't recognize. She stopped cleaning, cooking and caring. The tag line of her life was 'Pour me another drink.'

What a waste of a life.

When she doesn't come home at the time that she promised, my anxiety goes into overdrive. I turn around three times. Slap my face three times. Check the clock three times, on each visit to the kitchen. I do more things that I cannot talk about, I'm ashamed. I'm eaten up by worry.

She doesn't speak to auntie and uncle anymore and I'm so sad about this. I heard her argument on the phone. She was drunk as usual. She kept repeating that she did not make a racist remark about uncle Ali, that it was all a misunderstanding. Then she said that she hated him, because he wanted to keep auntie all to himself and that is why she had stopped coming to see us. After a few minutes of ranting, she said that she never wanted to see auntie again. Or the selfish Uncle Ali.

No one cried. I wished I could, but no tears came out. Instead, I punched my wall three times and broke a chair. Auntie was the only blood relative that mum had left, we needed her. Who was going to send me birthday and Christmas money now?

And I loved Uncle Ali. He sent me books on trees and cuttings from newspapers about environmental issues. He really cared about me.

I need mum to come to her senses. She tells dad on the phone that she never wants to be apart from him again, that when he gets out of jail, she wants us all to be a family. Me, him and her. Just like the old days. Then, when she puts down the receiver, she lies down in a huddle and cries like a baby. I put the pillow over my head and try to sleep but it's hard. I want to go over to her and comfort her, but I can't reach out like that, besides, it's her fault. She needs to grow up, smell the coffee. Behave like a proper parent.

I realize that in some ways, I'm lucky. She doesn't have a boyfriend. I mean, I could have a step father who is mean and nasty just like in the stories. Instead, I have a dad that I never see because he's banged up. They're divorced, but still she cries over him.

I'll never completely work people out.

So, I just think about trees.

Orangutans are going to be extinct soon, if we don't stop harvesting conflict palm oil from Borneo's tropical forests. Each time we chop down trees for the oil, these amazing furry creatures lose their habitats. Essentially, we're making them homeless and that is just not fair. Some companies make a lot of money using palm oil, so they don't care about where orangutans would sleep, they say that a lot of snack foods would not taste so good if they didn't use palm oil, beauty products would not be as effective. I read a lot about this, I like that they call it 'conflict palm oil' as if the oil comes from a source that they are at war with. Well, palm trees do not want to be chopped down for their oil, even if it is just so our shampoo is silkier than usual or our crisps crispier.

So, I say no to deforestation and no to the use of conflict palm oil in our snacks and products. I'm going to create a PowerPoint about it and show it to my IT teacher, maybe he can help me do something about it. That's another teacher who likes me, he says that my work is amazing. It's probably since I attend IT club after school and go over and over my work until it's polished and perfect. I love working with computers, that's my cup of tea, my bag. Computers don't make you upset, they just help you get things done. I wish I had one at home. I wish a lot of things...

Chapter 6

Ever since he was in primary school, Alan had to use his wits to survive. Well, we all do, don't we? It's called being sensible, like crossing the road at a pedestrian crossing when the lights show a green man, not just darting across the middle of the road. But in Alan's case, there were life skills like budgeting, cooking, cleaning and caring for his parents that he had to carry out singlehandedly. With his father in and out of prison from a very young age, he had been forced to step up. What a responsibility on the young, scrawny child! But they had lived in a two-bed house then, things had been different, nicer. His mum had missed his dad when he was inside, in jail. Each time he'd come out, she would blossom like a flower. She'd wash, dress in bright colours, sing as she cleaned the house and cook delicious meals. Then, after a few months or weeks sometimes, he'd be arrested again, and things would get bad again. For days, she would lie around crying. Then, she'd collect her benefits money and head straight to the pub. But Alan had started to sense when things were good and when they got bad. He had started to become rather crafty. Sometimes, he had to sneak ten or twenty pounds from her pocket when she was asleep. Other times, he was extra helpful on benefit collection days and she would take him with her to the post office where she would slip him money from the pile that she received.

Usually, he could get quite a lot for ten pounds if he focused on supermarket own brands. He'd get for example, a pack of baking potatoes, margarine, baked beans, bread, chocolate spread, cereal, milk, teabags and bananas. They'd all be the cheapest possible products of course, the ones without fancy names or packaging, but it meant that he was able to have dinner every night of the week. But, there had been many times when he didn't have food, when he felt so hungry that he felt sick. The one free meal that he was given, during term time at school, was not enough and, in the evenings, his stomach would growl with hunger pangs. Sometimes when this happened, he would knock on Mrs. Oyenusi's door, she lived two doors away and had often shown the boy kindness before. She was making jollof rice one day and saw him hanging around outside looking sad. Straight away, she'd called him in and offered him a large bowl of the red rice with vegetables which he'd devoured, it was delicious! After that, he knew that she had a warm heart and that he could, if needed ask for help.

But who wants to be a nuisance? So, he'd tried to be independent, or, putting it differently, he tried not to show his pain.

Then, the tragedy happened, and his mother was gone. His father had come out of prison, (he wished he hadn't), and they had been forced to move. The Housing Association had offered them a once only opportunity to have a fresh start in a 'good' area near a 'good' school, but it was a one bed flat far away from Mrs. Oyenusi. When he said 'apartment' it sounded better but really, it was a narrow, dirty flat with bare floorboards, peeling wallpaper and kitchen cupboards that hung loose. You had to walk through the kitchen to get to the bathroom which he didn't like, but then at least they had a roof over their heads, unlike homeless people that he saw huddled on the streets.

The man from the housing association had said that they could decorate the flat according to their tastes. They could, for example paint it, or put up new wallpaper, fix the cupboards and put down carpets. Alan could see that the man had a vision, the way he spoke. It was as if he was offering them a dream. There'd be father and son trips to DIY shops, the radio would be on while they both decorated the place, they'd stop for cups of tea but then carry on afterwards until it was all finished. After having hot baths, they'd get dressed in their good, clean clothes and pop to the shops to get takeaways as a reward for all that hard work.

But that had only been a brief, fleeting image, an impossible dream if you like. The reality was very very different. Alan's father did not like him. He called him a snitch or a goodie two shoes. He took the one bedroom for himself, leaving Alan to sleep on the flea infested sofa in the living room, that way Alan could watch the telly all night, he said with an evil smirk.

But when the social worker visited, her face was grim when she looked around. He had to block his ears as the conversation between her and his father became heated. It was Alan who had to have the bedroom, he was a child after all. He also had to be given pocket money and his father had a duty to cook and clean. She said that she would check, from time to time.

After that, things changed. He moved into the narrow bedroom with the single bed, bare floors and white cupboard. He had no telly in there, no game console. Just an old, embarrassing phone and charity shop books that he had bought himself, with bits of money, over time. He wondered if Uncle Ali continued to send him books and interesting bits of information, he wouldn't know the new address so maybe he was sending it to the old address. But he couldn't go to the old house, it was too far away. The thought of his presents sitting unloved in the post office back there made him so anxious that he had to clap his hands over his ears to block out noise and just think of the number three non-stop.

His books were precious. They wanted to be with him, not in the unclaimed section of the post office.

All his books were on one topic. Trees.

You see, Alan was passionate about trees. It was his number one hobby. Trees, for Alan, were more than just beautiful living things, they were higher beings with a life of their own, they were his spirit guides that he looked up to and depended on. The trunks were arteries, the sap was blood. A tree that was sliced or damaged would weep and bleed, he knew this by researching the bloodwood tree whose sap was blood red and even coagulated, like human blood. Cutting down trees made them cry or scream in agony, he couldn't bear it. It was one of the things that made him so angry that he wanted to lash out at woodcutters.

Sleeping was his second hobby. When he slept, he could dream, and dreams could take him to places that he would never ever be able to visit, in real life. Restaurants and supermarkets. Banquets. Feasts. He was hungry often now, because despite making promises to the social worker, his father never cooked or bought food for him and the cupboards were only used to store more stolen goods or bottles of alcohol. But if he went to bed hungry, he could conjure up feasts in his dreams. So, sleep was a priority. It kind of fed him. You never had to remind Alan about his bedtime. He would willingly go to bed, sometimes he slept at silly hours like six or seven pm. Then, he would melt into dreamworld.

Besides food, his favourite dream was about lost in an enchanted forest, surrounded by trees.

Trees would always remain his special subject, in fact he had a connection or a kinship that no one else would ever understand and he wouldn't want to discuss it anyway. People can be cruel. Especially other kids. He knew this from experience.

'Alan Arbour have you been to the harbour?' they sang.

'Alan Arbour wants to be a barber.'

There were worse taunts. Some picked up on his clothes, his hygiene, his looks, his seemingly lack of skills. His Special Needs.

Trees saved him from this constant bullying, gave him something else to focus on. And it was interesting how he was introduced to the subject in the first place. It almost felt like it was meant to be, like a connection that was meant to happen.

Alan

Chapter 7

It was a Thursday afternoon, and everyone had been collected from school. Except me. I could see that Miss was looking at her watch and getting edgy. Earlier, she'd been pleasant when I helped her to tidy the classroom but now, she kept interrogating me about why mum had not shown up to collect me. She said that she had called home a dozen times. I could have told her that she was wasting her time, we hadn't paid the bill and the phone was cut off. But I kept my mouth shut.

I was an inconvenience, a nuisance. She wanted to go home, put her feet up, pour that glass of wine, think of nothing. I heard her talking to Sir in the corridor, but I pretended like I wasn't listening, and I just concentrated on sweeping the dirt up.

Then, suddenly, I spotted a familiar black and white striped headscarf. Mariam! She lived a few doors away from us. She always arrived late to pick up her son Hussein as he played football after school. I ran towards her and hugged her long dress.

'Please take me with you, please! Pretty please!' I practically begged her. And she did, much to the delight of the teacher who promptly locked the classroom door and ran to her car, before Mariam changed her mind.

At home, I let myself in as usual and braced myself. Mum had been late before, lots and lots of times. But the way she was that morning, the way she'd been crying lately. It was worrying. It was as if I wasn't there. She'd clutched the picture of dad and her on their wedding day and sobbed into it non-stop, you'd think that they were not divorced or something.

'I'm sorry that it's your wedding anniversary,' I said softly. 'Do you want to go for a walk in the park?'

'Do I what?' Her eyes had been bleary.

Later, she kept laughing in between crying, saying how is a walk in the park going to bring back my husband?

Then, without warning, she left home, and the door banged shut. Silence. First, I thought that she'd made a mistake, that she'd been waiting for me to get ready for school and the door had closed by accident. But when I opened it, I saw that she wasn't there and when I looked out of the window I saw her walking determinedly away, wearing a smart black dress and red shoes, swinging her handbag as she moved.

I had to ask Mariam to take me to school. As we walked, she pulled out snacks from her bag: warm flatbread, olives, nuts. I stuffed it all into my mouth greedily. What a change from boring cereal! I treasured her warmth and support, but at the back of my mind, questions kept popping up like adverts on telly.

Where did mum go? Would she be back by the afternoon?

In the dinner hall, the cook saw my sad face and dished up a bigger than usual portion of chips and chicken for me, with a pudding of sponge cake and custard. I ate the lot in silence, but I still couldn't get the thoughts out of my mind. Half way through dinner, I started to well up and my salty tears dripped into my food as I shovelled it into my mouth.

Chapter 8

In year three, when he was about seven, a new teacher joined the school. She was to be his class teacher.

'Buongiorno,' she greeted them, her brown eyes twinkling. 'My name is Miss Pellegrini, I'm from Italy,' she said. 'I'm so looking forward to teaching you, it's my first time in the UK.'

His teacher from the previous year had been a lifeless, drab woman, who had criticized him for every small mistake. She would wander around the class with those sharp detective eyes looking like a cat about to pounce on prey. Everything that he did was wrong, and he ended up doing the tasks again and again, as correction. He'd ended up hating school. She refused to give him a part in the school play and had sat him apart from the others as he was slow and difficult to teach. She had also asked each child to bring in something from home for 'show and tell' and that's when he started kicking the walls. Didn't she know? What did he have at home that would be of interest to the other 'normal' kids? They'd make him a laughing stock. He could feel the way her eyes bore into him with hatred and his whole body drooped with shame when he entered her class.

But this new, vibrant teacher seemed passionate about helping all students and his eyes lit up a little now, when coming into the room. In the first week, when all the others had dashed out during break, Alan had sat there quietly, his head on the desk. Silence. It was so peaceful suddenly.

'Alan,' she crouched in front of him. 'Are you okay? You should be out in the fresh air, playing. Or eating.'

'It's okay Miss, I don't have friends. I will be fine just here.' He said sadly.

She thought for a minute, looking at him. Then, she said, 'Come, follow me.' She led him to the canteen.

'Miss, he only gets a free meal at lunch time,' a dinner lady said. 'It's break now, he has to wait.'

'I know,' said his teacher. 'That's why I'm getting two packs of sandwiches and two bottles of water.'

She was sharing her snack with him, Alan loved her already.

'You know Alan, I love nature,' she said when they had sat down under the large oak tree on the playground, to eat. 'I love the use of the fallen trees here because they provide great climbing structures for kids to play and interact with nature. That's why I liked you straightaway. What a name you have!'

The boy was enjoying the crisp, autumn breeze under the majestic tree. He had finished his cheese sandwich in a few large bites and was feeling happy, with his stomach full now. He noticed the gold and orange tinted leaves and the ancient, gnarled trunk. Yes, Miss was right, nature was so special. Sitting there made him feel peaceful even though the playful shouts of the other children filled the air. But now she was mentioning his name, what was she on about? Alan Arbour. There was nothing special about it. He frowned, confused.

'Do you not know what your surname means?' she asked. 'An arbour is a sheltered place in the garden where the sides and roof are formed by trees. An arboretum is a garden with many types of trees. On the twenty sixth of April, the UK and other countries celebrate Arbour Day, a holiday when people get together and plant trees. See, you *are* special. You have a special connection with trees.

You should use that. I know that sometimes things are not easy for you, but you can reach out and get help. Speak to me, speak to the Principal, we are here to support you. And there is no harm in hugging trees!'

Alan was smiling when he finished school that day. He had a collection of books under his arm that Miss had lent him. He would go home and go through each one. It was official. He had finally found a new hobby.

Alan

Chapter 9

I walked everywhere. I went to the pub three times and waited outside for thirty minutes. She wasn't there. I kept running back home to check if she'd returned but she hadn't. I did this, eleven times and this made me really anxious, everything was supposed to be in threes. I hate eleven. I just do.

I went into the post office, the Co-op, the Polish mini-market, the six off licenses, and then I just walked around the area, looking in bins, in alleys, even in people's gardens.

I called her name until my voice was raw in my throat.

After about six hours, I saw some legs sticking out, under a pile of rubbish with those famous red shoes of hers. Exhausted but desperate, I pulled her onto her side. Her dark hair was matted and stinky with vomit and alcohol, her handbag was empty, the gold clasp broken off. She looked like she was just sleeping. But she was dead. I know because she wasn't breathing.

I was nine years old.

I knew that everything would change if I went to the police, so I didn't do anything just yet. I just sat on the pavement next to the body, watching over her, letting the tears flow. Later, I went back to the flat and cried myself to sleep.

The next morning, I went into the police station.

'My mum's dead,' I said in a small voice.

Then, everything happened quickly.

Chapter 10

Birthday list: Shoes/trainers. My shoes are broken. It's embarrassing.

Al x

It was his thirteenth birthday and he had written the message on an empty cornflakes box. Then, he placed it on the cracked kitchen work top, hoping that his dad would notice the writing in bold red, on the white top half of the box. He'd stolen the red marker pen from school, along with some other things. He had to. It was true, other kids teased him more now that his socks were peeping out of the front of one shoe. He didn't even want a game or a console, which is pretty much what everyone wanted, he just wanted shoes. It had rained, and his wet socks and shoes had made a slush slush sound, in the corridor. Someone had pointed, and everyone had laughed.

He hoped there would be something that evening. Cake would be perfect. The librarian had been the only one who knew, he'd gotten to know Miss Williams well because of his constant use of the library when no wanted him in lessons. 'Here's wishing you a very happy birthday,' she'd announced when he was there. She'd given him a badge saying 'Bookworm' as well as a fully stocked pencil case and a bookmark. All had pictures of trees as Miss knew him well. He tried not to cry when accepting it, but later, when he was all alone in the bathroom, he didn't stop the tears flowing. Miss Williams was an angel, she was his champion.

That afternoon, he skipped home despite the shoe problem. As he approached the landing outside his flat, he stopped and sniffed the air the way a bear would at the hint of a delicious meal cooking indoors. Cautiously, his stomach growling now, he opened the door. Something had happened to his dad.

He was singing. He had had a haircut, a bath and had put on new clothes and deodorant. The flat was spotlessly clean and there were candles and fresh flowers on the small table in the living room. From the kitchen, there came the sound of something bubbling away and the delicious smell tingled his nostrils. His dad had remembered! He was going to have a party after all!

He bounded into the kitchen and threw himself against his dad, pressing himself so close that he could smell his fresh, recently showered smell. 'Oi watch it mate! I just changed my clothes!' His father scolded but he was smiling. 'Listen, I've got something for you,' he said.

Shoes. Thank you, thank you, thank you.

'You're the best!' he gushed.

He glanced inside the large pan. 'Chili con carne?' he asked, glancing at the cooked rice and salad on the side.

'Correct,' said dad.'

'Can't wait to try,' he said, reaching for a spoon.

The aroma of spices, garlic and minced meat made him ravenous, he could hardly wait for dinner. But suddenly, the spoon was being slapped away from him and he was being made to hand over the tin of kidney beans from a shopping bag on the side, instead. Inside, nestled a clear plastic pouch holding four cupcakes with pale, creamy swirls, some blue, some pink. He took them out carefully after handing over the beans. He would place them on the old dining room table, napkins would be nice amongst the flowers, candles and cake but it was okay, his dad had made a huge effort here and he could forgive him for forgetting to buy them.

Then, he stopped in his tracks.

'Put them back! They're not for you.'

'What?' he hadn't heard properly, it happened sometimes when he was concentrating on something so intently, he could drown out the voices of others.

'Put the cakes back! Now!' his dad barked the orders as a fine sweat broke out onto his forehead. 'I have a date tonight, I'm making her dinner. If you can be a good boy by disappearing for the night, you know, get out of our way, that would be much appreciated.' He gave a wink and reached into his jeans. Two one-pound coins fell out. 'Here you go, go get chips or something. Just give us a bit of space okay?' Another wink.

'Dad, where do you want me to go?' He asked this in a small voice, his bottom lip trembling as it did just before he started to cry. He must not show his dad how he felt. No never! Not now!

'I don't know where fifteen-year old's go! Anywhere. Go for a sleepover with your mates. Whatever.'

'I'm not fifteen, I'm thirteen. Today.'

'Ughhh huh. Sorry, you're in my way.' He was trying to reach the cupboard where a dismal array of hardened, unused spices sat on the shelf, sticky with dirt.

'What is it boy? I asked you to go. Didn't I? Surely you can give your old man a break sometimes.'

'Dad, it's my birthday.'

'Oh, right.' He dug into his pockets. A two‑pound coin fell out. 'Go have fun for a change!' he urged.

'I have Asperger's. I have no friends. I've been bullied all my life. Why don't you know this?'

He didn't say it of course. Instead, tears stinging his eyes, he shrugged on his coat, which was worn so thin that the insides had been torn away, the zip was touch and go, sometimes, it let him down and failed to work. He emptied his school bag, folded a thin blanket on the end of his bed and stuffed it into his bag, then added a few pairs of cheap socks that he'd had for years, a school jumper, and the four pounds. Wordlessly, he stepped into the hallway where his old bike lay propped against the wall. If only he could have it fixed. If only.... tears streaming down his face now, he walked out, closing the door behind him.

Alan

Chapter 11

I had a swarm of services around me. First, I was taken on a train to Hampshire by a social worker who bought me a burger, chips and a milkshake. She kept saying that I should cry and 'let it all out,' but I said that I didn't want to do that. Instead, I wanted to know whether auntie Linda would meet us at the station where the social worker would hand me over. Or would she take me all the way to her house? I loved that house, even though I had only been there once, a long, long time ago.

Even more exciting, was that Hampshire is where the glorious New Forest is. Now that, is part of dreams, I can assure you. The sight of those ponies, grazing in that unspoilt way, the little streams and brooks, the woodland. It's got everything. You could be lost there just in exploring. It's always been on my bucket list and now, I had my chance! Of course, I had to ask auntie nicely about taking me there, I didn't want to overload her, she had just lost her only sister. But the social worker said that she had hinted on the phone to auntie, that taking me there would be therapeutic, something to aid my recovery from the trauma. So, it was likely that I would get to go. I had to be careful, she advised. No doing things in threes. Well, maybe in my room. No arguing or kicking things. I had my ten steps to calm down, in my bag. I had to use it. We were lucky that she had accepted me as Uncle Ali was poorly, and she had a lot on her hands right now.

I had to be well behaved, constantly. When I did start school, it would probably be one of those units, not a proper school. After all, I found my mum, dead. And I hadn't cried much. I needed a supportive space to come to terms with my new situation in my own time, and mainstream school was not a huge priority right now. Those units were small and had specially trained staff to help me cope with grief. Usually, they were for kids who had been kicked out of mainstream school for behaviour issues. But sometimes, you got other kids in there too. Kids like me.

Then, the social worker told me her name and punched her number into the new smartphone that she handed me, just in case I needed something and wanted to contact her. I pocketed the phone but clapped my hands over my ears as she went on and on. It was too much. I just wanted to look out of the window and enjoy the scenery in silence. If she wouldn't stop talking, I would maybe throw a tantrum. So, I told her that.

Then, when she had shut up, I pulled out the phone. I googled:

THE NEW FOREST

and immediately, the screaming voices in my head stopped.

Chapter 12

February is the coldest month, who had said that? Was it from a poem that a teacher had read out? Or just a weather report? He wasn't sure, but he felt it now as he stepped out into the street. He needed a place to sit down, to rest, huddle perhaps, to escape the biting cold. The idea of the hot chips that would have tempted him at other times, faded into insignificance now. He couldn't eat properly when he was upset. It was a pity that he didn't live on the edge of a forest, Epping Forest, say. Life would have been easy then, he could simply head out and get lost in the warm arms of nature. Even in February, it would welcome him, it would not be cold. He could trust trees, they were not unkind or cruel, or selfish. They reached out to him, saying, 'Come and rest. We understand.'

The closest park was about a twenty-minute walk from the block of council flats where he lived, but he set out, determined. It was the only thing that would calm him now.

Darkness sets in early, in winter. He was lucky there was no snow, it was a clear but sharply cold night. He shivered as he walked, his gloveless hands would be pale and frozen if he hadn't stuffed them into his coat pockets. There were no children out that night. In fact, everything looked eerily quiet. Shopkeepers were beginning to pull down the awnings of shop fronts as it was past closing time, there was the butcher, the baker, the funeral parlour, the Co-op. No, the Co-op would be open until late. Maybe he could get something in there, later. He slouched past, looking and not looking, trying hard to forget the scene at the flat, his dad, blunt and insensitive, asking him to go away on his thirteenth birthday.

He could forgive many things. But he couldn't and wouldn't forgive that.

It was seven in the evening, when he finally got to the park. Under the street lamps, the benches looked as eerie as the trees, on this side of the park. It was as if the lights had picked out the benches in sharp relief. The other entrance had kid's stuff, swings, a see saw, a slide. There were some pretty flowers in freshly dug beds, in the spring. Pansies, daffodils, marigolds. But this far side where he was now, was the beginning of woodland. Thin, tall columns of young silver birch rose up from the long, matted grass, their creamy white barks slashed by grey and black cuts where the bark peeled off. They looked like eyes, staring spookily at him. He laid out his blanket on the cold, wooden bench and sat down. He'd have to sleep here for the night, hugging himself for warmth, using his schoolbag as a pillow. If it hadn't been so cold, it would be a pleasure, he thought. Just the reassuring sight of the elegant, narrow trees in their dazzling, snowy whiteness, silent and sharp, set off in the day by the milky white sky, pleased him. Happiness lit up his heart just thinking about it. He picked out the carpet of bluebells under the trees, the cluster of sparkling snowdrops.

My eyes are bleeding with the beauty of nature, he thought.

He was welling up.

When the sun came through in the morning, even a weak sun, it would cast a golden light, like a scene touched by something magical. He would see the wildflowers then. He was so wrapped up in his imagination that he didn't flinch when he saw the unicorn up ahead, making its way towards him.

I wish I could paint this scene, he thought. I want to capture it on paper, set it down. Or photograph it. I never want to leave this magical place. I would rather be amongst the sounds of nature, than the sounds of the city with the noise from traffic, shouty people, police sirens. Kids teasing and taunting.

Everything happens for a reason.

Suddenly, he was glad that he had been forced to leave his flat. Even the unicorn approaching, crashing through the forest towards him, did not concern him, he welcomed it. Although, he would have expected a unicorn to glide gracefully, or float. He watched it carefully, his heart singing with joy. Who would have thought that his life would have turned out to be such a fairytale? One minute, he was being miserable, another, magical things were being conjured out of thin air. For every second that he'd ever been unhappy, there'd be another that gave him pure, irrepressible joy. It bubbled and gurgled inside of him and he found himself not only smiling but laughing. It was the trees. The trees had given him this. With their silent approval and support of him, their love.

Of course, it wasn't a unicorn, and really Alan needed to check his eyesight as he may have needed glasses to accurately identify things in the distance. Instead, it was an old man with a long white beard. And no, he wasn't some forest creature out to rescue him, Alan realized, half amused, half curious. His name was Jim, he too liked to sleep on the bench, when he had fallen out with the staff at the homeless shelter. He had a sleeping bag, sandwiches and a flask full of hot tea that he'd bought in a café. Alan thought that he was surprisingly well prepared for spending a wintery night under the stars.

At first, they sat there on opposite ends, shivering in a stony silence.

What are you doing here? I was here first?

Alan had heard about dodgy people in parks. Even those with kind faces could turn out to be strange and cruel. But after breaking the ice by offering him tea, Jim proved to be an ally, a friend, not an enemy. He had left home years ago after having an argument with his father, something about not wanting to work as he suffered from depression. It had not gone down well with his father.

'No one understands me,' he chuckled, 'sometimes, I can hardly understand myself! It's better out here for me. There are no bills to pay, no house to manage, no one to nag me about getting a job when they know full well that I have a mental illness! I'm free. When I feel like it, I go to the shelter, other times, I come here, or go wherever I want. I'm not going back home, ever!'

He wanted to hear Alan's story. But Alan was tight lipped.

After a few minutes, he relaxed and said that it was his thirteenth birthday, he'd wanted shoes, but he got kicked out of home as his father had a date. He showed Jim his broken shoes as evidence of why he had been angry. The sock, peeping out, was black and sodden where it had trailed along the floor as the shoe gaped open. He said that he wasn't cross anymore, being here was actually a gift. He loved trees. He loved the way that his birthday had turned out, in the end.

Well, what happened next was the stuff of fairy tales, at least for Alan. Jim had been shaking his head vigorously while Alan spoke about his birthday, about being dumped on the streets by his father, and about the state of his shoes.

'No, no, no,' he said through clenched teeth. 'I simply can't let this go on. You're only young. You have miles to walk, adventures to experience. Unlike me, I'm old.' The funny thing is that the more Alan looked at Jim closely, the more he realized that he wasn't that old. If he shaved off the beard, for example, just like in those makeover shows on TV, it would take years off his face. He wasn't wrinkly, and his brown eyes looked cheerful and twinkly. Now, Jim was taking off his own black trainers that looked worn but in good condition still, he handed the pair to Alan. What were the chances of that? Being handed his dream present, in a park, by a complete stranger. Surely, it wouldn't fit him, or would it? He was so desperate, he would have worn anything unbroken, even if he had to wear six pairs of socks to pad them out. As if in a daze and forgetting all about the freezing cold settling in even more now that darkness had properly descended, he whipped off his worn shoes and put on the trainers, they were perfect, maybe a tiny bit big but with socks, anything was possible.

It felt so good to be wearing a decent pair of shoes. He looked up at Jim, tears starting to sting again.

'What will you wear?'

'I can't wear yours,' he laughed, 'those are destined straight for the bin.' He pulled out a few things from his rucksack. At the bottom of the little pile, was a pair of old, worn shoes.

'At the shelter, we get given these donations, see! That's how I got those trainers. It's okay, I can wear my old ones for now. When I get back there tomorrow, I'll check the donation box for a better pair. Go on son, you take those!'

Son. When last had his father called him that and put love into the word? It had almost never happened. And here was a complete stranger reaching out to him, helping him and showing that he cared. He had to be wary though. This was London and strange, dark things happened here sometimes, especially in parks. You had to have eyes at the back of your head to look out for yourself here. He liked Jim, but he would keep him at arm's length, until he knew more.

His thoughts flickered to his dad. Come to think of it, he had so many questions about him, he had put them all to the back of his mind to keep his sanity. But now, the questions reared up again. Was the man his real dad? Alan was genuinely not sure. For starters, the man seemed to hate him. Who, after being reminded that it was his son's thirteenth birthday, would still ask him to sleep out just because of a silly date? He'd been claiming benefits but never seemed to spend any on Alan. There was never any food at home, sometimes he would even forget to pay the electricity and gas and they'd have to use candles. How he'd survived in the last few years was indeed a miracle, he was worse off now than when his mother was alive.

His neighbours had helped when they saw him rummage through bins one day. Once a week, Mrs. Shen made him dinner and he'd collect it and eat it in his room. It was just the leftovers from her own dinner but still it was nutritious and delicious food. On the other side, a quiet, older man who didn't speak much English bought him groceries every now and then: tins of soup, bread, fruit. He accepted it all graciously. Sometimes, he would find money at home and then he'd head to the supermarket straight away. Somehow, he'd managed. At school he had a free meal every day. But thinking about it, he hadn't seen his dad for ages after he'd gone to prison. Then, after years, he'd come out after his mum died. Anything could have happened in that time, he knew that. People changed in their looks and in their hearts.

But this man wasn't his dad. He was sure of it.

Alan

Chapter 13

I don't want to play the disabled card, harping on and on about hypersensitivity and anxiety triggers.

I had simply run out of things to say.

Besides, my head was filled now, by images of the New Forest. So, I just watched and waited, all those days in auntie and uncle's gorgeous house. The first day, I was exhausted. After dinner, I had a bath and went straight to bed in my new pajamas. I noticed the bags of new clothes on the side, but I took no notice. Sleep was what I craved. I must have slept for ages. The following morning, I had to pinch myself, I really felt like I was still dreaming. Like I had stepped onto a film set where they were exploring the lives of the uber classy.

Rose jam with rose petals. The bewitching and sensual smells filled the room. Rose jam? I had never even heard of that. Strawberry or peach maybe but not that! What planet were these people on? She was spreading it on a buttered scone and quaffing champagne. I read something about the word 'quaff' once, it meant drinking something alcoholic in a way that you put your all into it. Mum used to knock the drinks back, hard, in small, quick movements. But auntie really relishes the taste, by rolling it around on her tongue. A small, elegant lady with creamy skin, shiny with health, a broad smile, bright, intelligent eyes. Her silky blonde hair in a neat French knot. She looked like a more sophisticated version of mum, before mum dyed her hair black. Life had been kind to her, even her two white poodles looked beautifully coiffed and healthy. Sitting there, in the sun-drenched conservatory with its generous wicker chairs and plump white cushions, I felt like I was in another world. One where people spoke softly, smiled sweetly, and moved with deft, confident movements. The inhabitants of this world moved forwards. Always. Surrounded by books, broadsheet newspapers, soft music, light laughter, china teapots and matching cups, tiered cake stands laden with small, tempting morsels: delicate finger sandwiches, tiny muffins and scones, the smallest squares of ultra rich cakes bursting with flavoured creams. The garnishes giving an aroma of their own: scattered rose petals, sprigs of fragrant thyme, basil leaves.

It felt like my world had been chalk, and this was cheese. Polar opposites. And yet, my mother and this vision of a woman had been related by blood! It was so hard to imagine.

No one spoke of what happened. They didn't force me to eat or drink, didn't try to get me out of my new pajamas. Nothing. The wheels of life just moved on.

Auntie was having brunch with her best friend, Alicia. She was a middle-aged Black woman with skin the colour of dark chocolate and a voice like tinkling piano keys. If I had thawed out, over the loss of mum, I would have liked her. But I felt frozen inside. And broken. In fact, I didn't think that I could ever be put back together after this. Maybe it was the final straw. The undoing of me. And, maybe that too, was a blessing. To join my mum wherever she was. I couldn't, I just couldn't carry on.

I gravitated towards uncle who was mooching about still in his silk dressing gown and pajamas, fussing over the dogs but doing nothing too tiring because of his heart problems. He'd aged so much since the last time I'd seen him, when I was a child. Fine lines marked his brown face now, white stubble sat stubbornly on his cheeks and chin, bruising me when he hugged me. After ignoring their invitation to help myself from the staggering array of food, I finally grabbed a plate and heaped it high enough to be embarrassed, then disappeared into the TV lounge where I sat on the recliner, in front of the impressive plasma while the hours passed.

Everyone whispered around me as soon as I exited the conservatory. Should we ask him to? Do we think that he would want to? He doesn't look so good. He doesn't want to talk. Poor Alan. Bless him. There were phone calls about me, emails. More whispers and gossiping. Mostly they left me alone. I watched a lot of TV, read, ate a lot, and listened to uncle's stories about travel. He had been a globetrotter in his younger days, travelling the length and breadth of the globe. Sometimes, he just delivered a monologue, in that slow, droning voice of his but I just focused on the TV and drowned him out. The best thing was being allowed to have time off school. Or that unit, whatever.

A week passed. Like a robot, I put on the new clothes they had got me, used my smartphone just to set it up, took long baths in the impressive stand-alone tub, walked the dogs and ate non -stop as if I was making up for lost time. I didn't speak much, there was nothing to say. I was in shut down. Even when the dogs playfully bit my ankles, I let them get on with it. They all watched me carefully, auntie ruffled my hair complimenting me on my new haircut, when she passed me. Uncle tried to engage me by taking me shopping for books and comics, but my heart was not into it. Even when he gifted me with a shiny new silver laptop, I merely shrugged and walked off, leaving it on the dining table. I slept and slept and slept.

Then, one day, I came downstairs as usual and discovered that we were going to the New Forest for the day.

Chapter 14

Jim was a chatterbox. He said that he had experienced many problems since coming to the UK twenty years ago, as a refugee. His name was Julian spelled with an X as in Xiulian, but he pretended to be Jim just to blend in. He had had a family once, a mum and a dad just like Alan. His mum had died and his dad had not stopped nagging him to go to college or get a job and he had walked out, with nothing to his name. He waved Alan away when he wanted more information. That was all he was prepared to say about his parents. He was not an unhappy man. And he was not ungrateful for all the support that he received. He had the shelter, donations, and free, simple meals at the shelter when he was there. Sometimes of course, he wasn't there, like tonight. Space, the open air, moonlight, hugging trees, feeding birds. They were important to Jim. He couldn't explain it, it just was. Sleeping indoors was safe yes sure, but it disconnected him from nature, he said. When he slept out, he felt that rare thing that other homeless friends of his never mentioned.

Joy.

Alan was learning new words. Disconnected. Was that what he felt now that his mum was dead, and he felt no ties with anyone, in the whole world? Was it a connection that he was searching for when he roamed around in the forests, whispering to trees? He wished suddenly that he was connected to Jim, not his dad. For Jim, was like him. Maybe he too had a Special Need and had trouble reading and writing but he'd never admit something like that. Who would? Alan could understand that. Why would you shout it out to the rooftops when you would only get bullied, teased, picked on or physically hurt? Other people who didn't have it didn't always understand it.

'Own your diversity,' he'd heard a support assistant say once. 'Be proud of who you are!'

But why would you own something that others used to exclude you? It didn't make sense. Hiding it was better, helped you survive.

'Jim,' he said in a small voice, 'May I ask you for a big favour? I mean another favour, as you helped me with the shoe problem.' As Jim nodded, he went on, 'Could I stay with you please? Like could you be my forever dad from now on? I need you...' and his voice tailed off as he burst into great, noisy sobs.

Jim was crying too. 'Come here, you. Of course, I'm here for you. There's nothing that I wouldn't do to help any child. But you do already have a dad Alan. Remember that! And he'll be waiting for you in the morning.'

After polishing off Jim's food supplies, Alan slept in the sleeping bag, spread out on the bench. Jim said that he preferred the floor where he made himself comfortable using his heavy coat and blanket. It wasn't easy. All night, Alan kept waking to find the stars blinking at him in the dark sky. There must have been nocturnal animals, birds and creepy crawlies too he realized, though this had not troubled him with the seemingly gigantic body of Jim sound asleep on the grass next to his bench. The white trees silhouetted now in the moonlight looked truly spectacular and part of him wanted to stay up and hold that memory forever. But they whispered to him to sleep and rest and so he did.

In the morning, Jim walked him to his flat and he said goodbye reluctantly. They swopped phone numbers and Jim promised to check in on him. With his heart hammering loudly, he opened the door.

Alan had been diagnosed as having Special Needs from his first year at primary school. For nine whole years, he had received extra help from school, to enable him to learn. Some teachers called it support, some called it intervention. Sometimes, someone sat with him going over the basics like phonics and times tables over and over again, sometimes it took the form of putting his timetable together but in picture form, on large laminated card, one for the classroom and one to put on his wall at home. As we know, some teachers assigned him to the library and called that support as he was free to use the computers in a way that was not stressful or anxiety producing. Once, a brilliant support teacher had given him a laminated ten step programme to keep at home that, she said, could change his life forever if he kept it up.

At the time, he'd been prone to kick against doors and pull displays off the walls. If he was having a 'bad' day, he'd tip the table over and tear up as many books as he could. Students hated him more when he did this, and teachers would say, 'I want him out!' when they radioed for urgent help from the senior management team. He had spent a fair few days being out of lessons on the punishment desk in the Principal's office. So, he had nothing to lose but to go along with what the brilliant support teacher came up with. It said:

Self Help Strategies for Alan Arbour

1. Breath work: breathe deeply from the pit of your stomach or into it.

2. Be calm.

3. Say to myself: I can do this. It will be okay.

4. Use humour where possible. Jokes make the situation less tense.

5. Count slowly from 1 to 10. Decide if it's worth saying. Then, say it politely.

6. Avoid needing to get the last word in.

7. Try to understand the other person's/people's perspectives.

8. Think about changing something to lighten the mood/improve the situation.

9. Do not try to steal the show. Allow others to speak.

10. Walk away from the situation, get a drink of water or use the Time Out card, if this helps.

Later, he realised that she should have added:

11. Share information about your needs. For example, say 'I have a sensory overload issue, I can only deal with one thing at a time.'

12. Avoid monologues. Turn taking is the key to effective communication. This really was linked to number 9, but it was important so he would have given it its own space.

But he knew that it was important to her to stick to ten steps. Maybe she thought that he could only cope with the number ten. Or maybe it was her who was fixated on this number. It was always just the number three for Alan. She had got him to practise the ten steps with her and then, to memorise them.

The words were etched into Alan's mind.

But that morning, he did not feel like using them.

He burst into the living room, noticing that his dad was still in bed on the sofa bed pullout. He marched into the kitchen. The chilli sat in bowls atop rice, it had been largely untouched, and flies were buzzing excitedly around it now. The place was a mess. Two cakes had been thrown at the wall, the blue icing drying in sad patches while the crumbled remains decorated the floor. The stench of alcohol and food going bad made him want to be sick.

'What happened?' he demanded.

'I made it too spicy. And then, I added way too much salt for her liking. She didn't want it, we had an argument and she walked out!' His dad looked sad.

So, he could have given Alan a bit of the food the night before, he could have given him a cake, he could, he really could have made a bit of an effort.

Because he'd made all this effort, for this mystery woman, for nothing! Something in him laughed, 'ha ha!'

But something snapped too.

'I need to talk to you,' he said icily.

'What?' his dad swivelled his head around to look at him properly. In the few years that he had parented as a single dad, his son had been a quiet, gentle presence in the flat, he had barely complained when things went wrong, preferring instead to lose himself amongst his many books about trees. Now, his tone was assertive, and it sounded wrong, like he was scolding him.

'Ever since you went to prison and we stopped seeing you,' he began, 'I've covered for you. I had to take care of mum when she started drinking, I had to take care of the house, cooking and cleaning, checking that the bills were paid etcetera etcetera. I didn't want to find my mum dead, no, not at the tender age of nine. But you came out of prison and I thought okay, everything happens for a reason, so I tried to get on with things.

But it hasn't worked, has it? I mean you do know that I have special needs, right? Dyslexia, dyspraxia, ADHD, Asperger's, you name it, I have it.' His dad nodded but seemed confused. Where had this come from? And where was it going?

'Well, you must know about my special needs cos you get extra money from the government for me correct?'

Silence. So, it was all about money???

'My question is, where is it? The money? The money you get for being a single parent? The money you get for raising a child who is special?'

His dad threw off the duvet and got to his feet. For a moment, sitting in the single armchair, Alan thought that he would strike him. His eyes flashed angrily, and he stared at his son.

But Alan wouldn't let up. 'The reason I'm asking is that every three months, the social worker meets me at school and asks if everything is okay. I always say yes, of course. But, it's not okay. And from now on, I want to tell her that I don't want to live with you anymore. Because,' and he pointed to his heart, 'inside here, *I'm* not okay. Yesterday was my thirteenth birthday. I asked you for just one thing, a pair of shoes, why? Cos my school shoes are broken, so broken that the few nice kids that don't bully me, are now laughing. I didn't ask for a games console like other boys, or a game, or a new phone, or a duvet cover, or a carpet to stop me getting caught on the nails in the bare floorboards. I just asked for a pair of shoes, trainers from the market would have been okay. But no, I didn't get that. I got kicked out of my own house, so I had to spend the night on a park bench in the woods, talking to a homeless man who thankfully, had the kindness to donate a pair of *his* shoes to me. All because he couldn't bear to see the state that I was in. You put me in danger by sending a thirteen-year-old child to sleep in a park, you're lucky nothing bad happened to me! Which parent does that? Do you love me? Do you? Have you ever loved me?'

At this point, Alan stopped. He remembered what he had written in his diary a long time ago. 'I like to cry sometimes. The salty tears tickle my face.' Now, he needed a cry. The tears that had threatened earlier came, hot and furious, so much so that for a few minutes he was completely blinded.

'I've been protecting people all my life. I turned a blind eye to mum's problems and look where she ended up. But I'm not doing that again, I'm not standing back and watching you descend into neglect and ruin. That's not fair to me! So, I'm not doing it anymore. I hate you!' he said. 'I asked a homeless man to be my forever daddy. He said yes. I don't want to live here anymore. Because living on the street now is preferable to living at so called home, where I am clearly not wanted! You can have a girlfriend every night if you want. I'm going.'

He hadn't counted to ten, he hadn't been careful about breathing. He hadn't used humour. He had simply lashed out, contrary to what he had been taught.

Then, he marched out of the living room, went straight into his own room and lay on the bed, sobbing.

Minutes passed. There was a stunned silence from the living room. Then, a knock on his bedroom door and his dad's voice, gentler now, 'Okay boy. You made some relevant points and I'm sorry. Wait here, I'm coming back.'

He opened the door and threw a roll of notes on the bed. The notes were rolled tight and held together by an elastic band, Alan heard the soft thud as it hit the bare floorboards.

Then, he heard the front door close with a soft click and there was silence.

Alan

Chapter 15

Money! At last! Why did I have to have a meltdown just to get money owed to me? I think quickly. It's a Saturday. Snow is forecast for tomorrow. I'm so sick of feeling cold.

I head across town to a cheap charity shop I saw once. Everything there was five pounds and under. I choose a thickly padded, thermal black coat with a hood, a V neck black jumper, a grey and white striped scarf and a pair of black jeans. Yay! Clothes at last! I ask if they sell socks and the old lady who works there gives me a suspicious look and moves painstakingly slowly to the back. Meanwhile, I take in the shop properly, choosing to ignore the sickly smells of dead people and disease. There are no hangers here, everything is piled high. The other shoppers are like me. People who like to rummage.

Some of them look homeless, there's a mother with a kid in a pram. Poverty is a kind of unspoken disease that we share, we avoid eye contact because this is not the kind of place for conversation, no one wants to admit defeat. None of us are high rollers or success stories. Besides, I'm an Aspie, no one expects eye contact from me.

The lady is back, she inches towards me with a large box containing unloved items, single socks, random ties, some underwear. She tells me that they are throwing it out, I can have it. I place all my precious packages carefully in a bin bag and leave. I paid next to nothing, but I have a whole new wardrobe there.

And it won't be a wardrobe malfunction as it's all black, people never get tired of black so for once, I'm on the road to acceptance. They can call me goth I don't give a fig. To wear clothes with no holes, in the British winter! Big thumbs up to that!

Next, I go into the Turkish barbers around the corner and ask for the latest, most fashionable cut. It's not expensive and I deserve to look good. It's still my birthday, in fact, it's my un-birthday. To me, that means that it's the day after my birthday. And I'm determined to celebrate it. I've always liked the idea of an un-birthday. To restrict yourself to just one day of celebrations, after waiting a whole year is just not fair. Anything can happen to ruin your special day. So, an un-birthday on the day after your birthday makes sense. That's why I'm determined to celebrate today.

Back in the flat, I give it a good clean which involves tidying the mess that dad made. Hopefully, he will notice. Hopefully he will see me as a good investment, now that we are on better terms and he has given me money. I must work quickly. I have a plan, it's an ode to Jim, my shoe saviour.

I never forget good deeds.

They say that needy people have problems reflecting gratitude, we over thank people. That's me. That's so me.

After meeting Jim in what feels like a sacred grove in the park, I know that I need to stay connected to this wonderful human being. To think that I've passed homeless beggars on the street and just thought that they were all druggies or dangerous. I want to take that back now, by something that no one would expect of an Aspie. I want to reach out and say thank you.

After mum died, I lived in a place that was neither dark nor light. I merely existed. Now, I had met a person who had broken me out of that fog.

I would never win a MasterChef competition. I don't have the advanced culinary skills or the imagination for that. So, I bought a bag of baking potatoes, some tins of beans and grated cheese. Good old British food! Hopefully, he'll like jacket potatoes with beans and cheese washed down with blackcurrant squash. For afters, I got an apple pie and squirty cream. I got a single birthday candle and placed it on the pie, I had to get paper plates too as ours are all chipped and embarrassing. I put credit onto my relic of a phone and called him, to invite him over. I'm so excited, I'm shaking. I've also put on my new jeans and jumper, I think that with my haircut I look quite handsome. I've even doused myself with dad's deodorant.

I haven't had many people in my corner. Jim is a good soul, I'm going to collect people like him. I'm going to be a magnet for light filled people who are capable of showing love.

I have two pounds left, and I don't care, I made a connection! Aspies have a hard time connecting. But I have worked on this. I feel euphoric, like I'm conquering my fears.

I feel this immense need to create a brand- new world. A world not defined by able people. A world that is soft and flowy and safe, that can accommodate edges, angles and the bit in between, where fun, laughter and love are more important than barriers, categories and hard definitions. I'm disappearing in this current situation, I've always been manipulated into being voiceless. And I don't think I'm being too ambitious by trying to create this 'brave, new world.' Lots of disabled people feel lost in our current reality simply because, as it stands, we are just an afterthought. Look at publicity school photos. There's the White kid, the Black kid, a girl and a boy. They won't include someone in a wheelchair or someone who looks odd. Despite the illusion of inclusion, we are excluded, we put people off. Only when key visitors come, then they roll us out. Then, I'm not relegated to the library anymore, like an invisible freak. They show me off and take credit for me, for how far I've come.

'Look at the slow learners, they can walk, talk and operate computers. We include them in everything that we do. We're a proper little community, at this school.'

Lies, lies, lies.

I wanted Jim to be true to who he is, but he still doesn't want to use his real name Xiulian, so I stopped nagging. He liked our simple, sparse flat. I think he even spruced himself up for the dinner. Maybe he was surprised that I bothered to call him, after all, I could have taken the shoes and disappeared. Most people do things like that. I told him my whole life story from cover to cover and he listened quietly and patiently, nursing the two tins of dad's beer that we found under the sofa. He hasn't told me off or patronized me by crying, he just says that life has been tough for us. And I agree.

When he leaves for the shelter, I'm happy for him that he's got somewhere. I'm relieved that he's okay. I tell him that it's dangerous on the streets. He really needs to get some qualifications and get a job. That way, he won't have to rely on donations, or food that's out of date, that he gets from supermarket bins. If he gets his own place, I can visit him. I know about his mental health issues, he has told me about his bouts of depression. I don't mind, I just want to help. I can clean his place and cook him some simple meals, like omelettes, jacket potatoes and pasta.

I don't want anything bad happening to Jim. Not only because he took my bike away to fix.

He's like family to me now.

He calls me the collector of kind souls.

Chapter 16

For three nights, he didn't see his dad.

Any other thirteen -year old would have had a meltdown, understandably, at the prospect of being left alone this much. But the poor, brave little boy had become accustomed to these hit and miss attempts at parenting, in fact, he had become so self- reliant that he didn't think much of it. It's against the law to leave a child alone like this, but in many ways the boy was past caring. He treasured his personal space, the silence hugged him like a comfort blanket. People around him liked him and had shown kindness and generosity by donating food. If he had to scrape the barrel so to speak, there was always the idea of raiding supermarket bins under cover of dark, where you could find whole packets of unused food. Jim had taught him a few survival tricks, like this. And of course, he now knew where to find Jim, his new forever father.

Mrs. Shen had knocked on his door and delivered a mouthwatering plate of steaming hot noodles, covered in some light sauce, with a separate bowl of beef strips and vegetables. Earlier, the kind gentleman from number six, had knocked on his door with a parcel containing a small carton of milk, sugar, tea bags and bread. When he gushed out a 'thank you so much!' the man had replied, 'No Eenglish.' The man had flashed him a smile showing startling white teeth in his gentle brown face. He was reaching out to Alan. A beautiful, old soul, Alan thought. I'm a magnet for kind souls.

Alan had thought deeply about the generosity of others, how his neighbours had constantly reached out to him, over the years. It had mellowed him, softened his character, so to speak. No longer was he angry and bitter. He had accepted them, these souls who had been drawn to helping him.

Without them, he would not have survived.

He vowed to return the help. One day.

On Wednesday morning, he heard the doorknob rattle while he was sitting calmly in the living room, eating cereal and reading a book, a weak early spring sun streaming in through the curtainless windows. In walked his dad. As usual, his clothes looked like they'd been slept in, in fact, his hair, skin and clothes reeked heavily of alcohol, sweat and cigarettes. But he hadn't stopped off to offer explanations or excuses about why he had neglected his son. First, he threw a new smartphone across to Alan by way of a birthday gift. Then, his eyes bright with suppressed excitement, he twirled a set of car keys in one hand. In the other, he clutched a black bin bag that seemed half full of something oblong as far as Alan could make out by the shape. Without talking his eyes off Alan, he issued his demands in short, crisp sentences.

'Pack a bag. Now. We're leaving in fifteen minutes. I have a car. Let's go.'

'Go? Where?' He'd been enjoying the peace and quiet, the stolen days off school that he had decided to take, as his dad hadn't been there to monitor him.

Then, 'I don't want to go anywhere.' The 'with you' part hung in the air, unsaid.

But his dad wasn't listening to his whiny, feeble voice.

'NOW!'

The stress etched on his white face made his eyes look extra mean and small. He dangled his car keys in front of Alan's nose as if to say see, we really do have a car now. Reluctantly, Alan reached for his schoolbag and packed his new things into it. He threw the coat on over his old trackie bottoms and hoodie that he'd used as pajamas and put on thick socks with his trainers. Meanwhile, he kept his beady eyes on his dad, as if by watching him, he would get answers as to what was happening and where they were going. First, his dad hauled the large black suitcase from behind the sofa and flicked off the thick dust stubbornly clinging onto it. Next, he ransacked the flat, flinging open cupboard doors, looking under the sofa, even removing loose floorboards to find little bundles of 'lost' items that he kissed as if he was being reunited with something precious that he'd lost. He stuffed these and his own meagre belongings into the case, still holding the black bin bag. Finally, he found a sheaf of paperwork and threw this and the black bag into the case. An old sleeping bag and blankets were piled on top.

So! They were going away! Was it a holiday? Or more likely, were they running away from the law? Alan thought quickly while his father was preoccupied, running a bath. His back was turned, the time to act was now!

Quick as a flash, he lifted the blankets, reached into the black bin bag and peered inside. Just as he thought. Money! Twenty- pound notes in bundles, tied together with paper bands, there must be what, a hundred there? He must have robbed a bank or a shop. Without thinking, he knew what he must do. He pulled out one bundle and counted it, his heart racing in his ribcage. Two thousand pounds. In his room, his row of books sat in a neat row on the single shelf. He selected a hardback with a glossy cover, untied the band and placed the notes in the middle of the book. Then, he wrote on the inside cover:

For you, Jim. To say thank you for saving me.

He closed the book, placed his house key on the top, shoved everything in a plastic bag and used the last of his precious tape to create a secure package which he handed to Mrs. Shen in the flat opposite, telling her in hushed tones that his friend Jim would come to fetch the parcel and that she was not to give it to anyone else. He shook her hand by way of thanks and said that he was off on holiday with his dad, but that his friend would come to stay, to keep an eye on things. Poor bewildered Mrs. Shen, she wanted to hug him, but she knew Alan's difficulties with that, his social awkwardness was etched on his little pale face already as if a panic attack was waiting to be unleashed. So, she simply nodded held his face and whispered, 'Be safe, I'll see you soon.'

Before he packed, he used the last of his credit on his old phone to text Jim to tell him to collect his parcel, and to offer him the flat to live in while they were away. Why not? Why shouldn't he be able to sleep in a bed, run a warm bath and cook food in the empty flat? His friendship with Jim was non-negotiable, he thought stubbornly. He would never give that up. Even if he was being kidnapped and made to go on the run with a known criminal.

Soon, they were in a Land Rover, speeding towards somewhere in the distance. Would they ever return? Or was this goodbye? As the engine purred to life, he craned his neck to take a final look at the grey pebble dashed building that had been disfigured by unsightly graffiti. It was hailed as 'urban' or 'street art' but he hated it, found it repulsive. Couldn't graffiti artists go and do it on their own homes instead of public buildings?' That way, they wouldn't force their so-called art on others. The pimply effect of the pebble dashed, concrete walls was enough to have to look at day in and day out, he thought. Then, to add the unpleasant words on it:

Immigrants get out! Brexit rules!
Go home foreigners!

There were other slurs too, written with questionable spelling that had made him furious. Imagine how unwelcome people felt when they saw it! Even if they just had to pass the building every day, the messages were hateful and offensive. They echoed the mean comments made by the bullies and other nasties at school and on the streets. But now, that he was leaving it all behind, he felt a pang of sadness. He had made memories here, good and bad, spent the last three years of his life here. And now, he was in a stolen car no doubt, speeding towards a prison sentence.

Alan felt curiously light headed. He'd always wanted to have a 4x4. Just to see what it felt like to be so elevated and yet so comfortable. He whipped out his new smartphone, even with no credit or Wi-Fi, he could still use it as a camera. He would take pictures of everything, the car, the journey, the trees on the way. He shifted on the cream leather seats at the back. He could spread out here and have a proper sleep. They had stopped at a petrol station and bought an alarming amount of sweets, crisps, chocolates, drinks and pre-made sandwiches. His dad had reached into the bin bag that he had stashed carefully in the suitcase, in the boot and removed a bundle of notes for this. He had winked at Alan as if to say, see we're co-conspirators in this criminal deed. And Alan had smiled, happy to finally be able to pick and choose his favourite sweets, stockpile them even. He could never be bored now. In the little petrol station shop, he had accepted anything his dad had suggested. There was phone credit for fifty pounds which he put onto his smartphone straight away, comics and magazines and a newspaper even though his reading was laboured and slow.

Back in the plushness of the car, he drank his hot chocolate even though it burnt his throat slightly and stuffed two boxes of chicken sandwiches down his throat, while his dad drank coffee, smoked cigarettes and fiddled with the radio. They were one day millionaires! It had been his mum's expression every time they collected money and spent it on the same day. And he was spending this money too, which meant that he was part of whatever this was. He could have called the police. But he didn't. He could have called Jim. But no. Maybe he was his father's son, maybe it ran in the family. Criminal. Jailbird. It was in his blood too, he could see it now. His grandfather on his dad's side had been an ex-con too, the same for his uncles. That was why his mum had refused to mix with that side of the family. But blood was thicker than water. And he was his father's son. Just one look at the pale skins, the shifty blue eyes, dark hair and skinny, long frames and you could tell. Of course, his dad had a low, squidgy pot belly now, and salt and pepper hair that was thinning in the front. But still. They were two peas in a pod. He too, had experienced learning difficulties at school but unlike Alan, he had given up. Alan would never give up. Future Alan was just a few years away, a world of photography or forest work awaited. It was a delicious thought, his new 'go to' these days.

He didn't want to overthink this, he really didn't. Because, as the car sped off away from London, he could feel a panic attack coming on now and there was no one trustworthy around to help him through it. Where was his Time Out card? Well, even if he found it he couldn't use it here. But he needed something.

Fresh air. Trees. He should have carried a sick bag. He needed to think.

For the first time, he looked at his dad closely. He had to climb into the passenger seat for this, but his dad had the radio on and seemed lost in his thoughts. Obviously, he had known and loved his dad during his childhood. But then there was the divorce and things dried up after that for a bit. When his dad went to prison, it spelled disaster for their relationship as his mum wouldn't take him on the visits, preferring to go alone. Now, it felt like time had skipped past those forgotten years and they were back together. Bandits in cahoots. Bonnie and Clyde. His dad had committed another robbery and the evidence was the money in the bin bag. He'd also probably stolen the Land Rover, it looked too smart, too sophisticated for someone like his dad to choose to buy it.

Prison. A young offender's institution. Alan had watched a presentation by an ex young criminal in which he had tried to deter the kids from choosing the wrong pathway. He'd shown slides of how horrible it was to be incarcerated twenty-four seven, how mean and nasty the other inmates were, and how he'd been terribly depressed inside. Now, on the outside, he'd turned his life around by working as a shining beacon of positivity to young people at risk of going off the rails. There'd been several kids like that at Alan's school. But Alan had never in a million years thought that that was him.

Now, all he could think of was bars, a narrow, cramped cell, a cellmate who was not sympathetic to his needs, eating disgusting slop and more taunting and bullying, unchecked this time. He would mock Alan, force him to change his ritual from his beloved three to maybe four or worse, two. And life would be an endless nightmare after that.

He couldn't bear it. And now, his dad had involved him in something unsavoury, something that would look like Alan was in it too. He'd definitely go to prison for this, if caught. Or maybe it was a case of when.

Alan

Chapter 17

I've really turned a corner. I had to. One of the support teachers told me that the government only helps you until you turn twenty -five. After that, you're on your own.

Everything that I have been through has been building up to get me where I want to be. Working in the woodlands, or a career as a landscape photographer. It's so exciting to have a goal, to be passionate about something. They say that I fixate on things, become obsessed. It's so true. I can't stop thinking about Future Alan. Alan, in ten years' time. I would have my own place and decorate it in a way that suited my personality. Trees. Oh yes, the pure joy of it! I would paint my flat green and have miniature trees in pots everywhere. All my tree books would be in elegant wooden bookcases along one wall. My sofas would be simple. Black.

Outside, in my garden, I would plant fruit trees, for example, the iconic British apple tree, maybe a peach and a plum as well. There'd be ornamental trees like the densely flowering cherry and, my all-time favourite tree, the magnolia, whose large, goblet shaped, pink flowers are scented with honey and lavender notes. They are also a symbol of a love of nature which sums me up perfectly. I would so love to plant the golden rain tree or laburnum, which has elegant chains of brilliant yellow flowers in clusters so intense that it appears to be raining flowers. Can you just imagine that! Pity, because all parts of the tree are poisonous. That means that it is a deal breaker for paranoid, socially anxious me. Still, there's just so much that future Alan has to look forward to.

My intervention teacher says that I have to live in the present and at that, I merely nod that I understand and accept this. But she doesn't have the first clue about the ugliness of my current life and I don't want to have to go over these details yet again. In my mind and heart, I'm thinking that Future Alan will live a positively satisfying life, I have this fixed now, in my head.

Aspies are not supposed to have positive, successful relationships. Social interaction is our main problem. We typically can't read expressions or emotions and therefore have trouble perceiving and making meaning. Often, we get things wrong. When I was younger, I lashed out at a charming Black support assistant who had done a lot for me, so it was grossly unfair to take my anger out on her. Without thinking it through, I made a mistake and called her a bad word. Straight away she dealt with it. She went through the whole scenario, once I'd calmed down, and explained in a very clear way, that the word was a racist term and that it was not acceptable to use it. She could have taken offense and reported it to the school as hate speech or bullying of a staff member. If it hadn't been her, say it happened to a member of the public, the person could have attacked me verbally or physically for being so offensive. I learned a lot, that day. She also worked with me about how to apologize and once I learnt the skill, I used it to say sorry to her.

In fact, I'm grateful that she has taught me about social situations via role play activities that she calls scripts. I refused to practise these embarrassing life lessons on how to handle people, in public, so we use a quiet room on the side of the library for this work. Each week, she brings up a potential situation, for example how to return a compliment or how to have a conversation with someone new. There are specific ones too like returning books to the library, ordering a meal, expressing dissatisfaction in a polite way, complaining about poor service, going shopping etcetera. Several of the situations are about reading and expressing emotions. She has role play cards and she plays Alan and I play the other character, then we switch. Every now and then, we stop to discuss teaching points. She says that these lessons are more important than learning how to read and write and I have to agree as they have helped me to interact more successfully.

I suppose I'm using these strategies with Jim. I'm actually attracting friends of my own accord! I can cross that milestone off my bucket list. Now to the next level. Finding a girlfriend.

Now that's going to be hard. Trouble is, there's no one that would want to be part of my life. Especially with the baggage I carry around.

Once, I said to a girl in my class that I fancied her. Her name was Jessica. She had long, split ended beetroot coloured hair and spidery lashes, thick with mascara. She was small, like a tree spirit, I imagined her with a crown of leaves and a dress made of white flowers, like the Queen of the Fairies, in 'A Midsummer Night's Dream'. She sniggered and asked me to repeat it, in front of her friends. All through break and lunch, I could see them talking about it. Then, after school, one of her minions came to deliver a message on a bit of paper.

'Meet me after school tomorrow, on the field by the weeping willow,' it said.

Can you imagine what I felt? I leapt up and punched the air, as if I'd scored a hattrick in the World Cup Football competition. She was one of the nicer girls, the type that didn't laugh at me or turn away in disgust, when I sat near her. To think that she was a few steps away from becoming my girlfriend!

The next day, I could hardly focus on anything and the day passed in a blur. A few times, I saw them in a cluster, laughing and pointing, but I ignored it and just focused on the meeting, after school. I'd showered in the morning and sprayed most of dad's deodorant on myself. I'd slicked my hair with his gel and bitten off the blackened rims of my nails. I was ready.

When the bell rang, I made a beeline to the tree, I stood under it for a while, then, I walked around it, then I sat under it, then I lay down, then, after waiting for five whole hours, I hugged the tree and wept with it.

She had played me for a fool.

Of course, she did not appear. Why would she? Teasing me in this way, was much more fun for her and her friends than actually having the bottle to get to know me.

Weeping willows have always fascinated me, their droopy shape symbolizing sadness. While they seem like a metaphor for anyone looking for healing, they are pretty flexible, adaptable trees whose branches can bend without snapping, that's why they use them to make baskets. Also, willows can grow in challenging conditions.

I was so heartbroken after that afternoon. I walked home, in the dark, feeling humiliated and sad. I knew that this would give the bullies fresh ammunition to tease me, in fact some kids seemed to come to school purely to poke fun at me. If I got angry enough, I could end up hurting someone. In primary school, I used to lash out at anything and once, I hurt a teacher. But in secondary school, I had come to my senses, grown up. What would be the point of assaulting the kids? There'd be harsh consequences here. Permanent exclusion maybe. They'd love to find a reason to kick me out to some dodgy behaviour unit reserved for kids with problems, and I didn't want that. I want to finish my schooling with success.

Still, the truth was that no one would go out with me, unlike the other boys with their arms around their girlfriends during the breaks and on the way home. No wonder they laughed at me. Loner, that's what I was.

I walked home in a thick pea soup of solitary aloneness, no one knew me, no one got me. I was fragmented, disconnected from everything except nature. I decided to take the long route home, through a lane thickly surrounded by wild, untamed hedges whose branches reached out and stabbed you with their sharp thorns. Then, I saw it. A rabbit quietly chewing, on a patch of grass, to the side. He watched me, I watched him. The world seemed to stop. And in that one moment, I suddenly knew that everything was going to be okay, that there was meaning to be found in unexpected places, if you were awake enough to look. I'd been walking around in a fog of disbelief, wallowing in my own misery, asleep. And I'd missed a bunch of magical moments.

That rabbit cushioned the blow that day. It was my soft landing from that potentially painful time.

So, I chose to take something positive from that afternoon. I chose to look again at that beautiful, graceful willow tree and I learned that through pain, we can develop and become stronger. And we can thrive and develop ourselves despite the odds. Maybe sending me to that tree was a blessing in a way, it made me stronger. I had challenging conditions just like the willow tree, if it could thrive then so could I.

I'm not a soldier. I'm just a damaged survivor in a fallen, defective world, trying desperately to hold on. Someone once said to me that showing my emotions was a sign of strength. I used to disagree thinking that if I opened up, I'd unleash that river that I've been holding back for so long. What if it wasn't possible to plug it back up? But I was willing to go along with the experiment. I started taking chances, I started opening up, I became more expressive, more honest, more confident.

Then, mum died.

That killed my interest in developing myself straight away.

In fact, I became more reclusive after that. I redefined broken. I was unput-together-able. Fragmented into jagged, nasty, splinters.

We'd lived in an area with rows upon rows of social housing. There was the complete absence of nature in the area, it was as if they had to sacrifice nature, to cater for us. And at that time, something deep inside me just yearned to be among trees, to hug their trunks, to gaze out at the emerald canopies. I had no relief from the pain, the constant, searing pain that bit and gnawed at my insides day in and day out. 'I'm starving for the chance to see trees, to be amongst nature, I hate this urban jungle.' I said to the social worker, when she asked how I was, after the funeral.

That was when they put me with auntie Linda and uncle Ali. And for a brief time, three weeks actually, I was beginning to thrive there, despite the odds. Then they let him out of jail.

Why? I will never know. Once a thief, always a thief. He had done his time, they said. He was a changed man. It was his human right to have his son back.

Really? Really?

Of course, he wanted to take care of his son, rekindle that bond that he'd missed. He knew they'd have to give him a council flat, money to start up, child benefit. And being a child with needs, he'd get extra money for me. So, I was his ticket to the land of milk and honey! But, when the leg up starter funds came, he invested in a few bits of tacky furniture from the charity shop and mysteriously, the funds dried up after that. Leopards never change their spots. Slowly but surely, he meddled again. The alcohol, cigarettes, petty crime. And a total neglect of me. How could I tell the social worker that she'd plucked me from a home where I had been loved and cared for, in favour of my so-called biological parent whose life was permanently on a downward spiral?

My lips were sealed. I was sick of sharing, or oversharing. Why not act like the recluse that I was supposed to be, I'm an Aspie after all?

Chapter 18

He was on the run with his dad.

'You should have seen this coming,' the voices said. His dad's criminal record and past behaviour should have given him clues. Damn. Why didn't he tell the social worker all this time? Maybe it was his fault after all. He had lied to her, deceived her. So, this was just and fair now.

They had left the town behind and now, the countryside welcomed them with its surreal beauty that Alan had always loved. On and on his dad drove, not making conversation, just sitting still and tight lipped, focusing on the road ahead or fiddling with the radio to find the mind-numbing tunes that he liked. Every now and again, he would ask for a fresh stick of gum, chewing got his mind off cigarettes. Traffic was thinning this time of the morning, in this direction, away from London. Earlier, he'd taken a picture of the sign saying 'Welcome to Essex' as he wanted to find out more about the history behind the three swords. He'd used his new phone to take other pictures of the landscape too, but each time, his dad had frowned and advised him not to. He never gave a reason, he just became increasingly moody and sulky each time the boy used his phone.

Then, they'd stopped off at another petrol station to check the tyres and he'd jumped out with relief, to use the bathroom. In the car, he had been focusing on a story that a teacher had read out, in primary school. It was the Hans Anderson fairy tale of 'Hansel and Gretel' where the two children had been abandoned in the forest by their father and his evil new wife, they had used a trail of breadcrumbs to find their way back home. He had been gripped by it, at the time. What if his mum had found an evil new husband who talked her into abandoning him somewhere? The forest would be a relief, but what if it was somewhere horrible, like a dodgy area in London known for knife crime attacks and gangs?' At the time, he went over and over the bit about the breadcrumbs until he knew it off by heart. And now, he knew that he had to leave a trail, in case the police and his social worker needed to find them. That way, he could explain that it wasn't him who committed the robbery, he hadn't pinched the car either.

In the bathroom, he used the marker pen that came free with the magazine to write on the mirror:

I'm Alan Arbour, I'm being kidnapped by a criminal. Please help! White Land Rover. Essex.

He would find the number of the nearest police station too and message them.

But back in the car, he couldn't find the phone. He had not left his phone in the bathroom or the shop, he knew this as he had placed it on the top of his bag which was on the back seat.

It was gone.

Waves of panic had started to wash over him, he had loved his phone. He must have dropped it when he got out. He must not mention it too much, maybe his dad was waiting to explode about how much it cost. He lay down on the seat, trying to sleep.

But he could still see out of the window. The town had melted into the countryside now, which filled him with happiness. Fields and farmland now replaced the housing estates. What charming, quaint scenes, he thought. How wonderful it would be to live in the isolated, colourful farmhouses dotted about on the landscape. What a pleasure it would be to look out onto golden bales of hay, laid out in straight lines, to be surrounded by a blanket of peace and quiet, away from the city. He closed his eyes for a bit, thinking about this and feeling heavy and tired suddenly, the tinkling background music, soft seats and purring of the car making sleep come easily.

When he woke up, all the farms had disappeared, because along the horizon, a thin blue line showed something that made him spring up in joy. The sea! They were nearing the sea. Alan had only gone to the seaside twice. Once when he was a small child with his mum and dad, and once when he was in primary school and classed as a 'severe behaviour problem,' along with five other special needs students. The inspectors had descended upon the school to check whether the students were learning or not, and suddenly, a support teacher had said that due to good behaviour, all six students would be rewarded with a trip out to the beach. They had been the complete opposite of good, they all knew that. But when inspectors came, the school wanted to showcase only the good kids, the high achievers. Kids who gave the school a bad name had to be shipped out for the day. Alan hated being invisible, but then who would refuse a trip out? Especially if it was free? There had been some fun moments, a ride on the Big Dipper that made his heart lurch, the carousel, the House of Horrors, and delicious fish and chips followed by ice cream and rock candy.

But his dad had suddenly turned difficult and strained. He had turned down the radio and was muttering about directions and the timing of the tides. He had pulled over and was looking at a timetable.

'Stop shouting!' he said, turning around to glare at the excited boy, 'sit down, NOW!'

'I wanna see the sea!' said Alan excitedly, ignoring his dad. If the child lock hadn't been on, he would have been out on the road, running recklessly to where he could get a good view.

'Drink this,' his dad said, handing him a soft drink, laced with some drops that he poured from a bottle in the glove box. Within ten minutes, Alan was fast asleep, leaving his dad to negotiate the detour that would take them off the mainland, towards the causeway across the Strood Channel, praying that the tide was not in so that he could cross swiftly and get to the meeting place on time.

Alan

Chapter 19

I'm probably dreaming but I can't get myself out of it.

I'm five years old. Mum is taking me to school super early, because they're trying out a new scheme, breakfast club. It's free for kids like me. She kisses me when she leaves me at the gate and I run in, my heart pounding. Will I ever see her again? Why do I always have to think like this? Why can't I trust?

As I sit down with my chocolate spread covered toast, a little girl approaches to sit opposite me.

'You've got the wrong colour jumper on,' she says. 'It's meant to be blue. Yours is green.'

I chew away, ignoring her.

'You're naughty. I saw you break the toys, the other day. Why do you do it?'

I'm listening but pretending to ignore her.

'I liked you at first,' she says. 'But now, I don't want you in my school. My mum says that kids like you are bad for the school.'

I look at her face carefully. If I throw the toast at her, I'd get chocolate all over her silly new jumper and that would be really funny. But it would also mean that I lose my breakfast, and I can't do that. I'm hungry. Always hungry. So, I just walk over to her side, snatch her muffin away from her and run away.

'Hey, I paid for that!' she says, crying.

By the time they've come to scold me, I've eaten it. I've also taken my stupid green jumper off and stuffed it in the bin. Mum knew that she had to get me a blue one, she knew. No one cares.

'You're a difficult young man Alan!'

'Don't care, don't care, don't care!'

I can't bear it, this trip down memory lane. I want to wake up.

Chapter 20

On the way to the New Forest National Park, the boy had had a setback, a turn.

A funeral procession passed them, a black carriage painted with purple lilies driven by two coachmen and two horses with coats as black as pitch. From the back seat of the car, he turned his head to watch, riveted, he even turned the windows down. Sensory underload was always preferable for Alan, to sensory overload. He was an Aspie. Quiet spaces, getting lost amongst non- demanding technology was always way more soothing than navigating the business of reading expressions and figuring out whose turn it was to speak. But now, he wanted to fill himself up with the sight, the smell, the sound, of the funeral taking place that day. He fixated on the horses, the purple ribbons on their tails swishing as they clop clopped on the cobbled street. A fleet of black cars followed, morose and solemn. He could make out a polished, richly presented coffin inside the carriage, when he craned his neck, he could make out gold handles and some kind of gold insignia on the sides. He imagined the scene at the cemetery, a loving family, dressed elegantly in shades of black, going weak at the knees in grief, the speeches poignant and sensitively delivered. Then white scented flowers thrown in with the coffin as it was lowered into the hole, Later, perhaps a tombstone with fancy, embossed calligraphy in gold. Maybe a big, posh one like an angel with wings.

Auntie crossed herself instinctively, taking her eyes off the steering wheel momentarily to glance around at the boy. He was staring so, so rudely. It was unnatural. But then, given his loss...auntie was lost for words. She had never expected to care for her estranged sister's son like this. She'd not wanted children for a reason. She'd always cherished her freedom, her space. It didn't mean that she didn't love him. But now, with him in perpetual mourning, under her skin every day, every night.

She didn't want this. The trip to the national park was an attempt to appease him, to bring him back. She wanted to wait and see. After all, she had uncle to focus on, his waning health.

Alan was still staring at the carriage, his head almost out of the window in consternation. He was looking at the colourful wreaths that decorated the carriage in gay commiseration. There were so many that they had to be tied to the sides, with wire. The middle one caught his eye and made him tear.

MUM

In creamy pink carnations. His mum's favourite flower. She'd loved the fullness and the frills of carnations. At the back of his mind, he thought:

My mother didn't have this. She had a pauper's burial with a cheap wooden closed coffin, within minutes of the vicar giving a speech, she was shoved into the oven and the flames of the furnace swallowed her up. I didn't get to say goodbye, I felt like I was on some Dickensian set, auditioning for a part in Oliver Twist. Except that this was real, not a performance. The year was 2018. I'll never ever forget it. As soon as I'm older, I'm getting a tattoo to mark the event and the date.

He said it in his head three times.

Then, he started wailing and screaming. He kicked at the car doors and tried to jump out of the window. Panicking, auntie pulled over and tried to talk him down, but it was no use. Finally, she put her arms around him while uncle drove the last few miles until they came to a sign that said:

NEW FOREST NATIONAL PARK. PLEASE DO NOT FEED THE PONIES.

Alan had dreamed of this from the very first time that he opened a book on 'Trees of Britain' which was in primary school. He let the tears dry on his face, blew his nose on auntie's tissue, and followed her after they parked. He had scratched her face when she had tried to comfort him, and he was hoping that she could forgive and forget.

Alan

Chapter 21

I woke up, feeling groggy and sluggish. I had been stretched out on the car seat and I had a pounding headache. I opened the door and got out on unsteady legs. The smell of the place was unfamiliar. It was earthy, and tangy and salty, we seemed to be near water. I liked it. Darkness had descended and the quiet was delicious. Dad was nowhere to be seen. The moon was out, and I could make out low buildings, a yacht club, a large gravelled courtyard area, a low wooden fence, a car park where our white Land Rover sat.

I pulled my hood up and zipped my jacket up tightly as I wandered around softly, not wanting to come up against anything scary or dangerous. But I was drawn to the smells of nature, there were huge trees dotted around, the air smelled fresh and farmish with the unmistakable salty tanginess of the sea nearby. I was curious. A country park near the sea? Where could this be? It had to be somewhere off the beaten track, for sure. That was why dad had chosen this hideout, it was deserted, and we could lie low for a while.

Trouble was, where were we exactly? I had to know if I was ever to get away from him. Clearly, no one had started looking for me despite my message. What a shame! I was starting to miss the place that I thought I dreaded the most: school. Clearly, I would be missed in school, the attendance officer would have been ringing home all week to get me to come in. I'd given a fictitious number at the start of the year, I couldn't quite put down that we had no phone or email, could I? Maybe she would report me to my social worker and that would alert her to the fact that I had been kidnapped. Maybe that would be the start of the hunt for me and later, they'd find my message on the petrol station toilet mirror. If only I had brought my old phone that I called the 'brick' as it was too big, bulky and embarrassing to use in public. I could have answered calls on it, Jim would have called to check on me. If I had it, I could have called Auntie Linda. But I wasn't sure if she was still talking to me after what happened in the New Forest that day. Come to think of it, it must have been easy for her to hand me over to my dad, when he got out of jail and wanted me to live with him. I'd shown myself up to be a handful.

In the silvery light of the moon, I sat at the base of a tree to think about Auntie Linda, I owed her an apology. Technically, I owed it to Uncle Ali too, except that he died a few months ago and I didn't even get to attend the funeral, dad refused to take me. All my people were leaving me, and I couldn't bear it. I put a card in the post, but I doubt she read it, probably saw my name and tore it up hastily. Who'd want to be associated with me, a tearaway, who was unpredictable, immature and always bound to give my handlers heart attacks?

I knew that the New Forest was home to ancient trees that were hundreds of years old. To me, they were more than beautifully shaped, living sculptures whose hollows and canopies provided habitats for a multitude of life forms. I saw them more like veterans or old age pensioners, doing their bit to support life. They had delivered a service to the ecosystem and even at their age, they had not stopped delivering. I wanted to hug them all to say thank you.

The woodland was full of birdsong that day, as I ran around looking for deer, grazing ponies, squirrels and any other animal I could find. It was late spring and the carpets of flowers, clear springs and golden light through the trees made me feel like I had finally come home. This was the place I'd been searching for all my life. I'd read about it and researched it, and I had finally reached it. So, my spirits soared when I got out of the car and ran into the forest. I could hear uncle shouting weakly behind me to be careful, he seemed to be aging right in front of me and the thought of him leaving us to join mum wherever she was, filled me with an anxiety so overwhelming that I would be physically sick if I allowed my mind to go there. As it was, tears were stinging my eyes as I ran, tears were never far away for me, they always threatened to embarrass me just when I tried to prove how capable and confident I was.

Behind me, I heard a loud crashing and I had to look. It was Auntie Linda, muttering to herself. 'Crazy for taking him in, what were we thinking? At our age, with all the responsibilities I have now.'

I'd stopped which gave her the chance to catch up with me.

'Alan!' she tried to control her voice, but it came across as shouting at me. 'Can't you see that uncle is really struggling with his health? Look, he can't even get out of the car, he has to sit there with a blanket, he's so weak! And you, you dash off like a wild animal, making me run after you. What are you thinking, carrying on like this? Your mum has passed, I know it's hard. But you need to get over yourself and deal with it. Don't become a menace to society just because you can't cope! Don't push good people away. Accept the help, accept the support. We love you. But I can't say that I've been impressed by you today!'

She had gripped my arm tightly in order to restrain me.

Something in me had snapped. It was all too much.

'Well, you can stop worrying about me, cos I won't be disturbing your posh lives anymore!' I screamed without thinking.

'Leave me alone! Just stop thinking that you can tell me what to do! I'm not coming back to your perfect house with your perfect husband and dogs and friends and food! I'm damaged goods. I'm not good enough for you!'

Then, I ran fast, sobbing, deep into the forest, trying to find a place to hide where she could never catch me, where no one could hurt me. I wanted desperately to feel safe, just for once!

'Alan! Come back!' she yelled, knowing that it was no use. To her, to the both, I had morphed from sensible Alan to strange, wild Alan who preferred going AWOL to having a relaxing day out with family. I could imagine how they'd react back in the car.

Why did we take him on, with all his many issues?

How can we handle someone like him, what with our health issues, our age?

How can we send him back and return to our normal lives?

I was not compatible with their uber sophisticated lives. Classical music, a five bedroomed detached house with an extensive, manicured garden, gourmet cuisine, designer everything. That was not me. Maybe I was meant for ghetto. Places where I could scream and cry and smash things without anyone blinking an eyelid. They'd see it as normal even. If I urinated on the stairs, dumped an old, stained mattress outside on the concrete play area or played loud music all day and night, they wouldn't care.

My head was too full of noise.

Or maybe I was the one who was broken and couldn't fit in anywhere.

But there, in the forest, at least I was finally free. There were no ifs or buts. I had found the perfect place to rest, recuperate, reflect, relax. All the R words to describe what I wanted and needed. When I finally stopped running, I found that I was in a clearing, far away from the beaten track. The little signposts were nowhere to be found, ahead of me was just grass fringed by trees, and the horizon of course. Exhausted, I lay down and went to sleep.

Chapter 22

The people who had promised to meet Alan's dad had not turned up. Everything had gone belly up. He saw now that he had been mistaken to bring the boy, to even dream of being able to create a life filled with adventure with him, to rewind the clock and start again, so to speak. Now, he had in his possession a stolen car and a bag full of stolen money. Maybe they were marked bills and the police were onto him already due to his lavish spending at the petrol station shops.

For once, just for once, he had tried to prove to his son that he could buy him whatever he wanted, that he could drive a decent car, take him on holiday. So many things had gone wrong for him, for them, this was his way of saying sorry to the boy. But it seemed now like his way of fixing their relationship only ended up damaging it even more and he couldn't bear that. He hadn't always been the dark and twisted individual that he knew Alan saw when he looked at him. Once, he had had a wife and a baby, a job, a house, a life. Then the accident and the illness. How it had changed everything for them, it was as if someone came in abruptly while you were listening to the most amazing song and switched off the stereo or threw it outside violently and unpredictably. In a heartbeat, he had lost everything that he had loved. After that, it was a case of surviving, existing. Sure, he had friends, but they were no gooders, criminal types that he could only class as slippery and sly. Instead of going away with them, he'd been left here to rot.

Surely, the police would be onto them by now. Any minute, they'd be here and then off he'd go back into prison. He was stupid, thinking that he could hide here. He'd come to Mersea Island as a child, had loved the estuary of the Colne and Blackwater rivers. The yacht club of West Mersea was where his own dad had taken him, there had been seafood suppers in restaurants on the marina, walks along with day trippers past white, weather boarded houses, banter with other fishermen, the tangy salt air on his face. He'd been fascinated by the snowy white seagulls, that had filled the sky with their strange screeches, he'd offered them his chips and the crafty birds had flocked around him, wanting more and more. His father had been the fisherman and had introduced him to his friends as 'my lad,' a term of endearment that he had secretly loved. Then, his father had gotten involved in something and had ended up in prison, his dreams of becoming a fisherman too had come crashing down.

Now, in the car park, he knew that he could never risk taking Alan to show him the marina. Too many people, too much attention. Not with Alan's social anxiety. No, they had to camp out here for a bit. Until he could straighten his thoughts. In his pocket, he touched the smartphone that he had given him and then taken away again. All those photos were clues as to where they were, how could he give them away like that? The young snake! He'd snatched it when he popped out to use the restroom, deleted the pictures and kept it. Better be safe than sorry. Besides, was Alan responsible enough to have a phone? Maybe not, it seemed.

He had taken a long, uneventful walk while he tried again and again to phone his friends. No answer. This was not the plan. How could they leave him in the lurch like this! Quick, he had to think. The Land Rover must have a tracking device, any minute, they'd be there, hunting them down. How to hide the money? The car? He'd have to go on foot, he could disappear quickly that way. Maybe make it to Wales, or Scotland. Maybe even France. Hide out there.

But Alan? With his constant questions and moaning, he had become a stone around his neck. He had always been that burden, too heavy to carry around. Better to travel light. That way, he could go rogue without answering to anyone.

Alan would be okay, he'd always be okay, he chuckled drily as he thought this. After all, he was highly intelligent with those special abilities that he'd been gifted with, and in the looks department he was a handsome little thing with his smooth bone white complexion, clear blue eyes and thick dark hair, especially now that he had had a fashionable haircut.

He could survive anywhere.

He would take him to the main road where he could hitch hike his way back to London. Or take him to the bus stop. Colchester town centre was only about forty -five minutes on the bus, he could get to the train station in no time, hop on a train and head for Stratford where he could either walk home or use the underground. He was a big, capable, clever boy. He'd used public transport on many occasions alone, and he could do it again, now. Then, he would disappear forever.

He walked back to the centre, his mind made up. Except that something was wrong. Alan was no longer asleep where he had left him, he had disappeared.

Alan

Chapter 23

An angel is dancing with me around a rainbow eucalyptus tree. I've always admired them, with their colourful, stripy, multicoloured bark bands. They look almost psychedelic, all those luminous colours. They could be on a fashion runway, with their decorated, elegant trunks that reminded me of mannequin's bodies. I never have to translate myself around trees. They get me. They feel me.

The angel is mum. A happy mum this time, not the woman who had gone to fat with her constant drinking and collapsing into bed. She has a silvery light running through her, with her hair loose and her chocolate eyes glowing, her presence lights up the whole of the New Forest.

'Mum, I miss you,' I whisper. 'I'm sorry you're gone!'

'I'm okay son,' she replies, ruffling my hair, smiling. 'I'm in a good place. Be happy now.'

Her voice is like music, and the notes have made their way into my soul. I love my mum so much, it's almost painful. I know that I was dreaming again somehow, that I had to wake up and make my way out again. But how could I make the dream end? I'd been waiting for this forever, this chance to reconnect with mum. To see her in this special place. To wake up would be to say goodbye to her, and I didn't want that.

'Take her with you, in your heart,' the tree whispered. 'Put her there, forever. But you must go back home now.'

I hug the trunk, relishing in the smooth, coldness of its skin, and slowly make my way back to the car park, using the white signposts as guidance.

'See?' I want to challenge my teachers, 'I *can* read. I can read signs.'

I'm so tempted to stray again; the forest is painfully beautiful. My heart stops with wonder and enchantment at the streams glistening in the soft evening light, the sound of crickets in the cool air, the thick, gnarled, tree roots that I almost stumble across, as my eyes are on stalks. I'm staring so hard at everything around me. I love the strange sculptures that trees make as they twist and turn, if you look hard enough, you can identify facial expressions in the bark, see the branches like fingers. They have such a powerful presence, if you watch carefully. In the summer, they would be in full leaf, some would break out into luminous flowers.

They whisper to me, 'Alan. Alan. Alan.'

For a moment I'm lost, drowning in the magic of the trees. Then, a higher purpose comes to me, something that I could be involved in, to help others.

I want to connect and support others with disability or special ability, whatever they want to call it. I want to share with others how nature has helped me. I want them to heal too.

'Whenever you feel down, find something to energize you. A walk in the park, barefoot on crisp leaves or on the soft grass underfoot. Hug trees for tactile, sensory support. Smell heavily perfumed flowers like lavender or visit a sensory garden. Better still, plant your own. Consider growing herbs, with their powerful scents. Whatever works, don't give up. We are special in so many ways, it's time to accept that and be part of society. Never, ever allow anyone to make you feel less of a person. Don't be voiceless. Have fun, laugh, be playful. Use your gifts in any way that works!'

Maybe I'll save that speech for a presentation at school. I have two requests that I want to put to the principal. One is this speech that I want to deliver to students with special needs. The other is that I want my school to be much more pro-active about celebrating Arbour day. Different classes could adopt specific trees, for example. We could go out and plant them in groups, in the school playground. We could invite the Woodland Trust to give presentations about their work, even Greenpeace could come in to inform us about endangered forests and ways in which we could all help. Our charity work could be more focused on preserving our woodlands.

Once, I watched a gardening programme about a talented, autistic guy who calls himself 'The Naked Gardener.' His passion for nature was so relatable that I was gripped, watching him transform gardens into havens of serenity and peace. I took a great deal away from the show, particularly the way in which he owned his autism and did not just brush it under the carpet. If we say that we appreciate diversity as a community, then accepting our special ability is the first step, I think.

Eventually, reluctantly, I end up in the car park, fully expecting the car not to be there. But my aunt and uncle have not abandoned me, even though it's late afternoon and they both look half asleep on the back seat. They don't make eye contact with me, they just give each other that look. As for me, I'm trying to pull it back, but it's a pathetic, feeble attempt, I know. I can't apologize enough for my outrageous behaviour. I don't want this lovely couple to see me as naughty or out of control. I explain politely that I'm trying to manage both my condition and what happened to my mum, but they wave my explanation away, they don't want to know. We drive back in stony silence.

Uncle takes his tablets as soon as we get in, and then he retreats to his room. Auntie disappears into the conservatory, with a cup of tea and her phone, no doubt, she's contacting the social worker. I'm shocked at the scratches on her face. My bad. I try to stave off the growing anxiety bubbling in me. What would happen now? I'd been trying to stop doing things in threes in order to break the habit, but seeing auntie's beautiful face marked like that, and the disbelief on her face when she spotted herself in the mirror makes me anxious enough to need to do something three times. I have to do something to say sorry.

Sorry.

Sorry.

Sorry.

I say it three times, in my head.

I make eight grilled cheese sandwiches whilst fighting the urge to make three, six or nine. I wash them down with several tall glasses of milk. I'm still buzzing with thoughts of that enchanted forest and the quaint, tumbling villages in the area. What a day out! But still, the realization that I made a major screw up sits uncomfortably with me. I really need to grow up and stop making these mistakes. If I don't want to end up like dad, I need to change things up urgently. I need just one more chance.

I spot the cheesecake in the fridge that auntie made to take to her friend. I love cheesecake, especially flavoured ones. Auntie's creation was just a dome of sweetened, soft cream cheese on a thick biscuit base, it lacks something, and I want to make it special. Carefully, I slide it out of the fridge and hold it on my flat, open palm to take a good look at it. What can I use to decorate it and say sorry at the same time? I try to rummage inside the fridge with my free hand searching for an ingredient that I can express my feelings with. I have a crazy feeling that something bad is going to happen, but I can't stop it. I'm a walking car crash.

Of course, it slips from my hand, bringing the cake down with a soft thud, the plate crashes into splinters.

Whaaaat!

Drama seems to follow me wherever I go. Voices around me and in my head, so loud I need to drown them out. I scream but no sound comes out! Aaaaaaaaagh!!! Why me, just when things are going so well?

'Sorry! Sorry! Sorry!'

But they've all gone to bed and no one's listening.

My anxiety has decided to kick in massively. My stomach is churning, and I'm flooded by crippling pain, a sweat has broken out on my neck and face, I can't breathe.

Make it go away, PLEASE! I have to practise my ten steps. Now! One, three, six, eight, nine, ten.

Okay.

My foot is bleeding. I leave the fridge door open and hobble away in search of a plaster.

Suddenly, I feel exhausted, so I curl up and sleep at the foot of the stairs.

Three difficult weeks later, they explain that I would be returning to London, to live with my dad who had come out of prison. From the chilly atmosphere in the house after the New Forest trip, who can say that it's a surprise?

Another move, another house, another experiment in supporting my needs. Welcome to Alan's messed up world!

Chapter 24

It had taken an hour to find Alan, pack up his things and put him on the bus with instructions on how to get home. He'd stuffed a thick roll of money into his bag and cried as he said goodbye. Then, he'd left without looking behind.

The boy had gritted his teeth at the thought of the trip alone. There would be strange people along the way, unfamiliar situations, like buying a train ticket for the correct train. But he had to try, he just had to. Because going back home and not being a fugitive from the law, is what he really wanted. He searched his mind for a bit of advice from an insanely helpful teacher:

'Where your fear is, there is your task,' he'd said. It was a quote from someone famous, but he couldn't remember now. It meant he had to face his fears, to grow and develop.

He had found his smartphone now, strangely it had been in his bag all along, but it had deleted all his pictures of his dad, the black bin bag and the route they had taken when they were running away. Still, he had his credit and could make calls. Once safely on the train to Stratford, he called Jim and explained the situation in high pitched, excited tones. They arranged to meet at Stratford Station.

He was fatherless now and there was something he wished to ask Jim. He didn't have a template to use for this, but who does? Technically, he wasn't an orphan as his dad was alive, somewhere. But he had gone rogue so that, to Alan counted as being dead.

'Jim,' he had asked, closing his eyes with hope. 'Will you adopt me? I want to be your son. I asked you before to be my forever father, remember? I meant it.'

The air was thick with tension. On the seat opposite, an old man with a milky eye shifted and stared, his small tongue hanging out loosely. Alan felt awkwardness creep up and grab him by the shoulders, his face reddened. The man watched him now, keen to find out the answer.

Please say yes.

Please say yes.

Please say yes.

'Alan, thank you for that money. I've been staying at your place and sorting myself out a bit. But something has happened. I wanted to tell you when you got here.' Jim's voice broke a little.

This was it. The moment when he refused politely and then, there would be the endless conveyor belt process of being passed from carer to carer, social worker to social worker.

'Don't worry! And thanks for nothing!' he shouted and ended the call. On the opposite seat, the man looked crestfallen. It was not the answer he had expected.

His phone was ringing. Alan ignored it. But it continued.

A little girl had left her mum on the seat diagonal to Alan, she indicated that she wanted to sit next to him and he reluctantly moved his bag aside for her.

'Are you going to answer that?' she asked. 'It's hurting my ears.'

Irritated, he accepted the call, rolling his eyes.

'The answer is yes! I'm going to do everything possible to adopt you, you rascal. You're going to have to listen to me and work with me. We both have issues to work on.'

Alan was crying. He nodded as if to say he accepted the challenge, even though Jim was on the phone and not in front of him.

Then, the shock.

'Alan, there's a lot to discuss my son. My father, he died last week. He's left the house to me. We're going to have to move and you'll never guess where it is...'

Alan

One year later

Chapter 25

I'm lying in my bedroom, my head resting on my forearms, relishing the fact that it's Sunday and I'm allowed to lie in as there's no school today. Usually, I spring out of bed at the crack of dawn, head for the shower, get dressed and make a beeline for the kitchen to start on breakfast. Jim and I are compatible house sharers, I make breakfast, he's in charge of dinner. Simple. But this morning, I want to reflect a little on this past year and how far we've come as a little family unit, I also want to take in my room and all my treasured possessions in it. Sometimes I want to pinch myself just to check if I'm awake or dreaming.

Jim gave me the largest room because I have more stuff than him and secretly, I think he wanted to say, 'Welcome Aboard, Son.' Being the only son, he'd inherited his father's little cottage on the outskirts of Epping Forest, he'd come into some money too. It took a lot of persuasion to get the council to allow a homeless man with a history of depression to adopt me, but between me, him, our lawyer and Mrs. Shen's witness statements, we convinced them that he was the best person for the job. Besides, mum's dead, dad's disappeared and auntie Linda, my only other relative, is poorly these days. There's also the fact that Jim isn't homeless anymore, far from it. He cleaned up his act almost overnight, as if adopting me was the push that he needed to sort himself out. Many moons ago, he used to be a carpenter, so I convinced him to open a workshop using the garage space, and now he makes bespoke furniture using reclaimed wood. It took him a good few months to set up, but nowadays, he turns out some truly unique, sought after pieces for high profile clients. He has an assistant helping him three days a week, as a support when he wants to kick back a bit and take time off, which is sensible.

Jim's depression, like my autism and other needs, will never go away. But together, we support each other and find ways to manage and move forward. Jim said that the council had caved in as they were struggling to cope with the number of vulnerable children in London. The system was buckling, he said. Something needed to give. So, we got our way in the end. I now have the forever father that I have always wanted.

As I look at my dark grey walls, wooden floors and black, patterned curtains, I know that this room suits me well and that even when I must leave home to attend university one day, I want to live at home and travel in. It took me such a long time to source the photo wallpaper of the forest along the one feature wall, and the huge desk that Jim made for me along the wall matches the bookcase that I found in an antique store. I've pretty much got everything here now. My books, the pictures I've taken with my new camera, my new clothes and my music. Even my duvet is grey, to match the colour scheme, I've landed on my feet here but I'm still an Aspie and I can't stand too much colour, or change.

Well, I had to compromise a tiny bit, because this house was just too far from my old school, even if I were to bike it every day. So, I had to go along with the flow when he said that he'd enroll me at the local secondary school, which is only a fifteen-minute bike ride away. My bike is superfast and sometimes, I can do it in ten. And again, lo and behold, I landed on my feet! This new school has given me the fresh start that I badly needed.

Over the holidays, I'd grown out my hair and had a fancy asymmetrical cut with some long bits, some short bits and even some purple bits. I wanted to match my hair with my new glasses which have purple frames, so I went a bit wild. Sometimes, I even paint my nails purple, and together with my new skinny jeans and black shirts, compliments my look, I think. The best bit was being chatted up in the photography class by this brainy new girl with black hair and skin the colour of my morning latte. She came over and introduced herself as Malika just as I was trying to figure out what my project would be called and before I knew it, she'd only gone and asked Miss if we could work together.

'It's wonderful to see you supporting other students, Alan,' said Miss. 'If you can hover around, sharing your expertise with the students that would be much appreciated.'

Excuse me? Expertise? I had blushed so much but then when they started coming up to ask questions, I really didn't have time to feel shy. I've titled my project 'Sacred Spaces,' which means that I can include groves, graveyards and odd pagan looking constructions that speak to me. Malika is a Maths wizard and has agreed to help me brush up on the subject if I did a quid pro quo and help her with photography. It involved lots of trips into the forest on our bikes to take pictures, although if I'm honest, some of those trips were just excuses to spend time with her. She's beautiful and thinks that I'm cool.

Cool? Me?

I punch the air often now. The most memorable was when she agreed to be my girlfriend, and when we went on our first outing date together, to the movies. Now, we see each other almost everyday after school, her parents think that I'm amazing and Jim, well he's just a big teddy bear, he loves it when I'm happy. We hang out in a small but steady group of friends, Malika and I. They're all a bit nerdy and they all have bikes, but they're my kind of people and it's just great to hang with kids who actually get me, even when we bike deep into the forest and hug trees.

The year has passed in such a whirlwind, but I'm so looking forward to Christmas, our first, in the house. Ever since I left Jim the message about Mrs. Shen and the money, they've become quite close friends. I know that she's single and I don't mind when she comes over for weekends to help him in the workshop or just to fuss over him. She's been a bit of a lifeline to me and now she's looking after us like we're family. She's doing some of the Christmas cooking but we're pitching in too, we do everything together these days. I'm planning to invite auntie Linda, Mrs. Oyenusi, Mariam and her family, Nicolai who used to gift me bags of shopping, my school friends, Malika and her parents and lastly, our new neighbours, Ben and Harry. Mrs. Shen says that she doesn't need an invitation as she will be staying for the week anyway.

I'll never forget what Jim used to call me: The collector of kind souls.

'It's as if people are drawn towards you,' he said.

It's true in a way, our house has become a meeting point for all the precious people in my life, who have reached out to me along the way. They've been beacons, lighting my way through the often challenging road that I have had to travel. And for that, I will be eternally grateful. There will always be room for them at our house and at our housewarming, I gave a speech that melted some of their hearts, so I know that they'll be keen to come again at Christmas and celebrate a truly multicultural kind of day. I have plans to make gratitude bags for each and every one, to say 'Thank you, for saving me.'

No one is perfect, I know that now. Even prime ministers make mistakes. Robots have glitches, computers crash. Parents go through unspeakable stress all over the world, I know because Jim and I talk about this often. That's why I'm so grateful to my mum and dad for giving it their best shot. I love them so much. As I grow older, I look in the mirror and see my dad staring at me, we look so similar it's uncanny. And mum's gentle presence guides me in my dreams. I know that she trusts Jim to be the mentor and soulmate that I needed, and I know that wherever she is, she is smiling. She would have turned thirty-six this December and we have plans to release thirty-six pink balloons in our back garden to remember her by. It's also a sign that I'm releasing myself from the grief that I've carried around for five whole years.

I need to move forward now. In two years, I will turn sixteen and school will be over. I need to think about college and university, I have so many plans.

But for now, I have everything I need.

The future Alan is here.

The end

Acknowledgements

I would like to thank the garden designer Alan Gardner aka the Autistic Gardener for allowing me to mention his work. His agent's website is factualmanagement.com

I would like to acknowledge the Woodlands Trust for all their fantastic conservation work and support for trees in the UK. Their website can be found at www.woodlandtrust.org.uk

I would like to thank Rainforest Action Network for the information on conflict palm oil and orangutans. They can be contacted on answers@ran.org

I would like to thank the Association of nature and Forest therapy at info@natureandforesttherapy.org for information on Shinrin Yoku.

About the Author

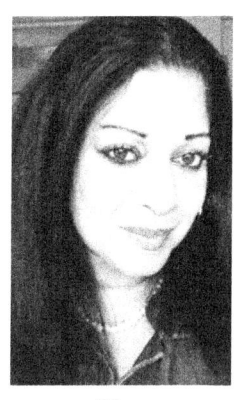

Sian Bezuidenhout

I was born in Durban, South Africa in 1964, to an Asian family during the heyday of the apartheid regime. Through writing stories as a child, I was transported to a land where I didn't have to worry about what was at times, a harsh reality, especially for someone who was not White.

I went on to study English Literature, Psychology and Drama, and later progressed to become the Head of Special Educational Needs departments in multiple schools. I have three daughters, and in between teaching English, I like to read and travel. I am currently doing an MA at Goldsmiths University, UK and this is my debut novel.

Printed in Great Britain
by Amazon